Approaches to High Throughput Toxicity Screening

Approaches to High Throughput Toxicity Screening

Edited by
C.K. Atterwill
P. Goldfarb and
W. Purcell

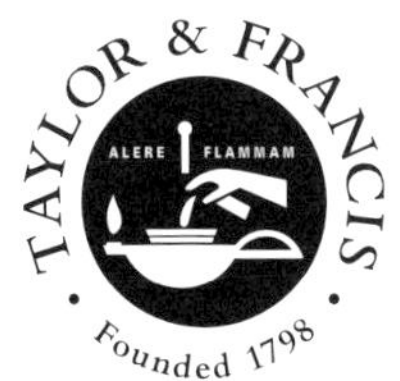

TAYLOR & FRANCIS
ALERE FLAMMAM
Founded 1798

First published 2000 by Taylor & Francis
11 New Fetter Lane, London EC4P 4EE

Simultaneously published in the USA and Canada
by Routledge 29 West 35th Street, New York, NY 10001

Taylor & Francis is an imprint of the Taylor & Francis Group

© 1999 Taylor & Francis Limited

Typeset in Melior by Graphicraft Limited, Hong Kong
Printed and bound in Great Britain by T.J. International,
Padstow, Cornwall

British Library Cataloguing in Publication Data
A catalogue record for this book is available from the British
Library

Library of Congress Cataloguing-in-Publication Data
Approaches to high throughput toxicity screening / [edited by]
C.K. Atterwill, P. Goldfarb, W. Purcell.
        p. cm.
    Includes bibliographical references and index.
    1. Toxicity testing—In vitro. 2. Drugs—Toxicology. I.
Atterwill, C.K. II. Purcell, W. (Wendy) III. Goldfarb, P. (Peter)
    RA1199.4.I5
    615'.1901—dc21   99-35680
                                                               CIP

ISBN 0-7484-0752-9

Contents

Preface

Toxicological or preclinical safety testing of new pharmaceutical medicines, using *in vitro* cell culture systems as animal alternatives, is an important and resurrected science. Alternative test systems have recently gained a higher profile owing to ethical, political, financial and scientific pressures as the drive to address seriously the 3 R's principle (Replacement, Refinement and Reduction of Animal Experimentation) gathers momentum. Over the last decade, and since the publication of the first *in vitro* toxicology textbook (Atterwill and Steele, 1987), we have seen new European validation bodies such as ECVAM (European Centre for the Validation of Alternative Methods) arise. Alongside this the UK Home Office APC (Animal Procedures Committee) have recently re-endorsed the 3R's strategy including alternative methodologies. Cosmetics testing for skin and eye irritancy has been restricted and viable *in vitro* alternatives now also exist.

A wealth of additional handbooks and protocols for *in vitro* toxicological methodologies has now been published, including O'Hare and Atterwill (1995), the Invitox protocols (FRAME) database, the BTS (British Toxicology Society) In Vitro Toxicology Working Party Report, numerous ECVAM workshop reports and more recently the ESTIV (European Society of Toxicology In Vitro) In Vitro Toxicology in Europe handbook (1998). Specific *in vitro* target organ toxicology textbooks are even appearing, such as those centred on very complex 'organs' such as the nervous system (Pentreath, 1999), not to mention a plethora of international conferences on preclinical lead optimization technologies.

The recent application of molecular biology (or toxicogenomics and proteomics) to toxicity testing will further enable a more accurate prediction of safety using *in vitro* systems and offers the potential for preclinical high throughput screening (HTS) systems. These can be automated to provide fast, cost-effective and more ethical approaches to toxicity screening in the preclinical lead optimization process of drug development.

Toxicogenomics is the study of organ and cellular responses to toxicity in terms of cellular stress gene induction and this new area is given wide coverage in this book. This family of genes (producing stress gene 'fingerprints') may in future allow more accurate prediction of human hazard at low doses of compounds using human cell-based systems (Rogers *et al.*, 1993). The recent development of gene expression microarrays (GEMs), *in situ* based assays for stress gene induction using gene-probes (e.g. scintillation proximity assays and reporter gene technology) combined with organotypic culture systems (e.g. liver and brain spheroid organ cultures) has and will enable automation and miniaturization of toxicogenomic-based high throughput screens in toxicology and drug metabolism. The approach will, across the pharmaceutical industry, lead to an integrated preclinical strategy incorporating predictive assays and databases for QSAR, genotoxicity, cellular and molecular toxicity, drug metabolism and pharmacokinetic profiling, solubility screening and drug absorption (via CACO-2 cell screens for GI permeability).

This book for the first time addresses an integrated approach to cellular and molecular toxicology and ADME screening using these new technologies and how they might be applied to the preclinical safety assessment and lead optimization of new pharmaceutical products in drug discovery.

References

Atterwill, C.K. and Steele, C.E., 1987, *In Vitro Methods in Toxicology*, Cambridge, UK: Cambridge University Press.

ESTIV, 1998, *In Vitro Toxicology in Europe: Final Report to the European Commission DGXI*, Paris, France: ESTIV.

O'Hare, S. and Atterwill, C.K., 1995, *In Vitro Toxicity Testing Protocols*, Humana Press.

Pentreath, V., 1999, *In Vitro Neurotoxicology*, London: Taylor & Francis.

Rogiers, V. *et al.*, 1993, *Human Cells in In Vitro Pharmacotoxicology*, Brussels: VUB Press.

1 Introduction

C.K. Atterwill, P. Goldfarb and W. Purcell (Editors)

Pharmaceutical research has been energized by the recent application of the concepts of combinatorial chemistry and molecular diversity to the discovery process. Designed to drastically reduce the amount of time and cost that is required for obtaining new bioactive compounds, one of the key features of this approach is the use of automation to more rapidly and efficiently generate, analyse, screen and optimize lead structures. Synthesis instrumentation has been the most challenging to develop owing to the stringent performance required. In particular, it needs to be capable of dealing with the wide variety of reaction conditions desired for small molecule library production, including temperature control, inert atmospheric provision and highly corrosive or active reagent handling, among others. Development of a series of robotic instruments, which are specifically designed for general synthetic applications, is key to this advance.

Alongside this revolution in chemistry, the explosive growth of genomics and proteomics in biology has fostered new and innovative thinking in the way that biologically relevant targets for drug discovery are identified, characterized and exploited. The interplay between molecular biology, protein biochemistry, robotics, miniaturization of assays, high throughput screening, chemo- and bio-informatics, libraries for screening and further biological and toxicological characterization of hits is crucial to pharmaceutical discovery and development programmes in the next decade (Figure 1.1). Here new endpoints and biomarkers in *in vitro* preclinical screening strategies (P.L.O.T. – Figure 1.1) will become increasingly important and supersede conventional *in vitro* tests (Figure 1.2). In a keynote address at an IBC's Drug Discovery Technology Congress (1997) in San Diego USA, Prof. George M Whitesides (Harvard University) described how the further transfer of technology from microelectronics into the fabrication of analytical and preparative microsystems offers an opportunity to increase throughput, flexibility and speed in lead discovery, lead optimization and drug development. New techniques were described, based on

Figure 1.1

Preclinical lead optimization technologies (P.L.O.T.) in drug development.

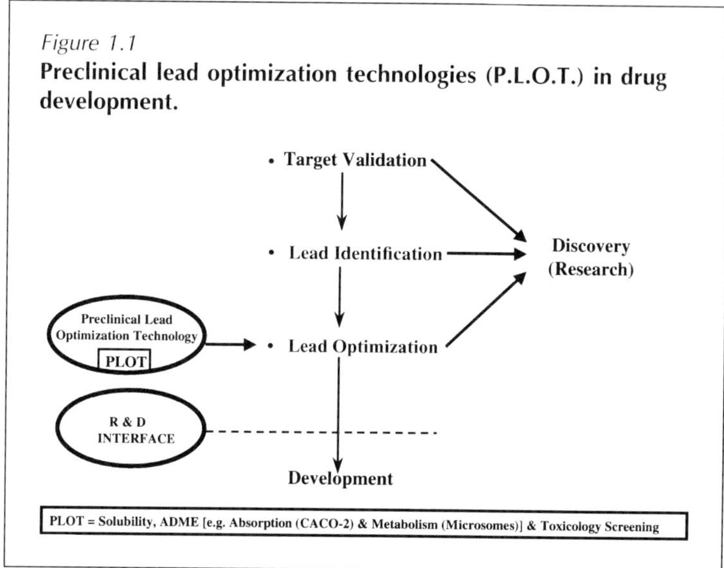

PLOT = Solubility, ADME [e.g. Absorption (CACO-2) & Metabolism (Microsomes)] & Toxicology Screening

Figure 1.2

General *in vitro* strategies.

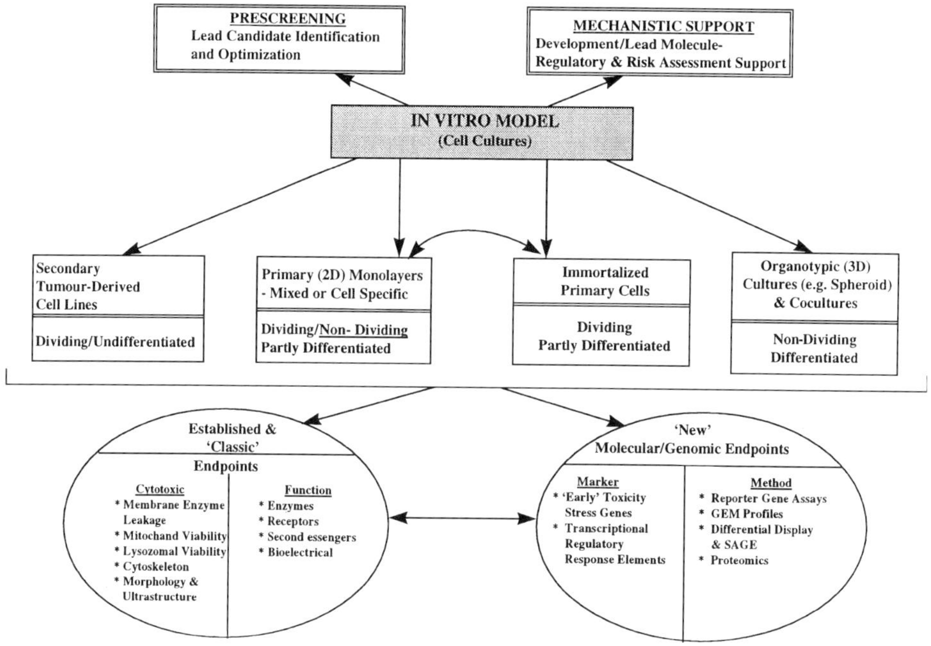

so-called 'soft lithography' that are better adapted than conventional photolithography to the problems in this area that require sophisticated chemical control of surfaces, ligands and cells. This type of advance could enable, for example, the growth of single cultured cells on microchip-based matrices for application of more sophisticated high throughput genomic technologies and chemical exposure.

The ability to pull out novel gene sequences from tissues in large numbers is now well established. However, the selection, characterization (including downstream biochemistry) and validation of the corresponding encoded proteins is just emerging. Understanding how these proteins are relevant to particular diseases and pathologies in drug safety requires the application of powerful robotics, bioinformatics and miniaturization technologies in order to cope with the numbers involved and to track the information obtained. The merging of the genomics and high throughput screening fields starts to offer answers to important questions about the isolated gene products. The final downstream, generally unknown, effects responsible for the compound's molecular toxicology profile lie in the protein domain and can be systematically observed and classified using Large Scale Biology's (LSB) ProGEx (proteomics technology for high throughput protein quantitation). Using this approach, LSB have developed a database of pharmaceutical gene regulation mechanisms useful in selection of drug candidates, analysis of toxicity, and in SAR studies of known and novel candidates.

Many of today's new targets have little precedent in terms of identifying compound leads. Consequently, developing new assay technologies to screen large libraries from chemical and biological sources is the only way to achieve and increase the throughput in numbers required to identify a hit. Once a hit is identified, new approaches to library design which integrate computer graphics and combinatorial chemistry using targeted libraries lead to rapid optimization. Automation is a key component of this process which ensures speed and efficiency, as is the early incorporation of absorption (bioavailability), metabolic, pharmacokinetic and toxicity data at the discovery stage of drug development called Preclinical Lead Optimization (Figure 1.2).

Affymetrix and Synteni's Gene Expression Micro-Arrays (GEMs) are widely used by leading-edge pharmaceutical, biotechnology and genomics companies for biological target discovery. GEMs can also provide an integrated framework for a parallel drug development process (Figures 1.3 and 1.4). GEMs containing thousands of human genes have generated significant quantitative data, as highlighted in Chapters 4

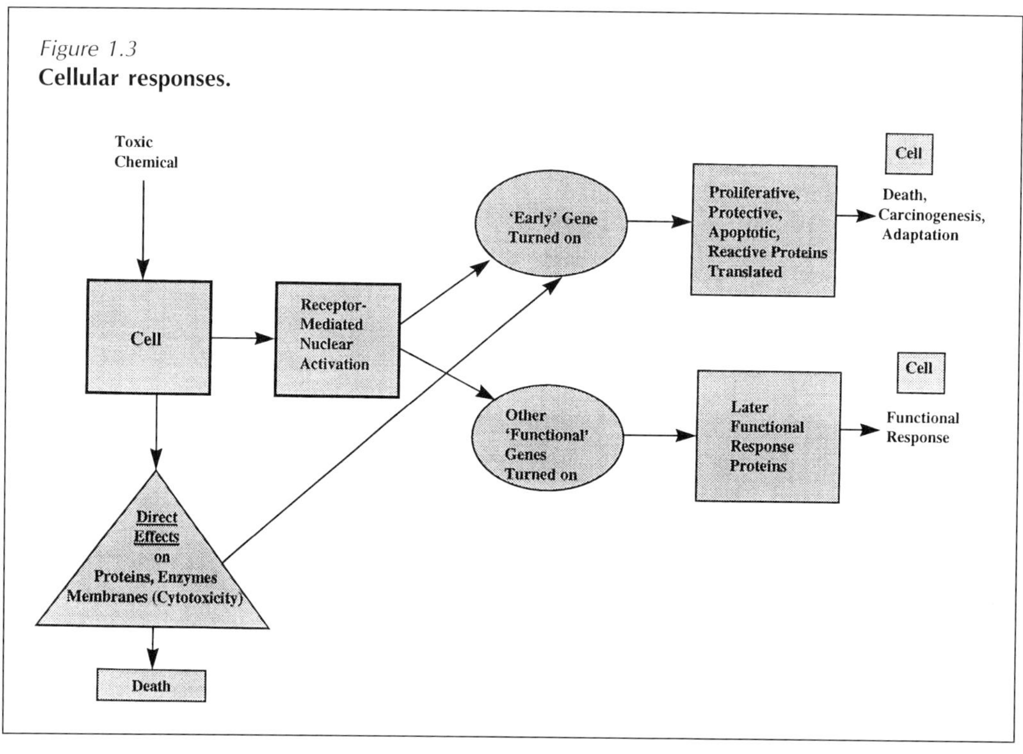

Figure 1.3
Cellular responses.

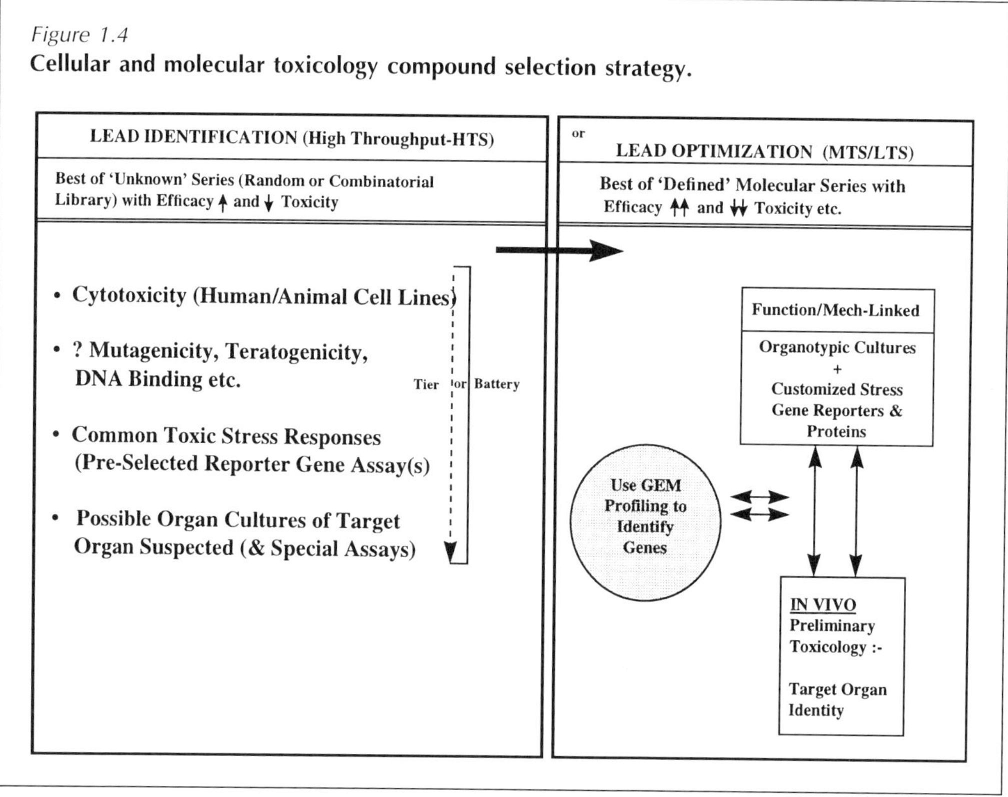

Figure 1.4
Cellular and molecular toxicology compound selection strategy.

and 5. The implications of this powerful new technology to the pharmaceutical industry are only just being realized. cDNA subtraction is a useful way to identify differentially expressed genes. However, current methods require large amounts of mRNA. Clontech have recently combined two technologies to facilitate cDNA subtraction from very small amounts of tissues. The first technology is an efficient method for generating high quality cDNA for sub-microgram quantities of total RNA called CapFinder. The second technology is an efficient PCR-based method for cDNA subtraction called Suppression Subtraction Hybridization. The Chiron Corporation have also developed bDNA technology for early toxicity assessment during the discovery programme. Branched DNA and Curagen technologies can be used for rapid quantitation of mRNA from tissues from standard or investigative toxicology studies. Branched assays are tailored to capture specific mRNA using custom-designed bDNA probes in lysates of cell lines or primary cultures of the target organ where the relationship between changes in gene expression and target organ toxicity can be evaluated. These findings from GEM and related technologies can be correlated with specific *in vivo* toxicity and pathology data (Figure 1.4). Adaptation to high throughput screening (HTS) allows an early approach for efficiently assessing toxicity at the discovery stage of drug development (Figure 1.5).

The discovery and development of new drugs directed against receptors and signal transduction pathways increasingly depends on functional medium and high throughput screening assays on living cells *in vitro*. This process passes through at least four stages, including:

- Identifying and functionally characterizing the target molecule
- Developing the cellular screening assay
- Running the cellular screen
- Functionally characterizing hits obtained from the cellular screen

Technical systems such as the Microphysiometer from Molecular Devices Inc. (for measuring cellular pH and metabolic changes related to receptor activation) and FLIPR (Fluorimetric Image Plate Reader – for measuring calcium fluxes and membrane potentials) are invaluable in this respect.

The flood of genomic data resulting from the Human Genome Project and other sequencing efforts are revealing a host of new molecular targets. Successful organizations will

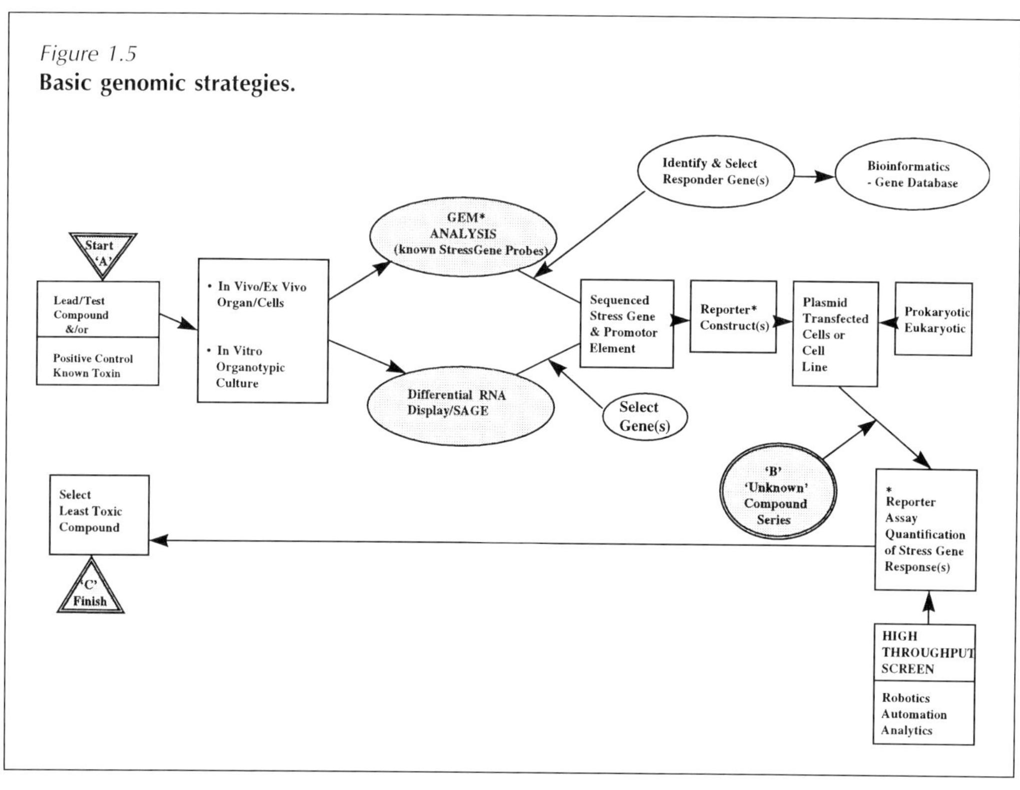

Figure 1.5
Basic genomic strategies.

be those that quickly identify and exploit targets with the best product potential.

Bioinformatics will exert considerable leverage on this whole process tools as the *in silico* technologies currently being developed by Incyte, i.e. LifeSeq® and ZooSeq® are amongst the first to appear. ZooSeq is the first commercial database to focus on genomic information on animal tissues from species currently used in preclinical toxicology and pharmacology studies. For example, by correlating a drug's effect in a rat with the animal's genetic makeup and then cross-referencing this data with LifeSeq's human gene sequence and expression database, this will enable better prediction of side effects in later clinical exposures.

Likewise, the Genie® and Bioglyphics® software recovery developed by Phase I Inc. and Molecular Dynamics enables the biological and quantitative significance of toxicological GEM profiles to be analysed and data to be stored and cross-matched in data warehouse files.

Lastly, to maximize fully the potential of these new technologies in preclinical toxicity screening, optimal organ-like culture systems are required that offer close functional, structural and metabolic similarity to the *in vivo* organs, as well as *in vitro* longevity. The appearance of the organ

Table 1.1 Technologies

	Pros	Cons
Gene expression microarrays (GEM)	No pre-selection of genes needed (in theory) can use normal cells and tissues for profiling	Costly to design and construct
Reporter genes	Easy to do assays	Not all control of expression is via promoter regions, needs undifferentiated cell lines/ immortalised cells. Costly to design and construct
Spheroid organotypic cultures	Multiple, interactive cell types. Longevity *in vitro*. Enables gene/protein profiling	Not applicable to every tissue yet

spheroid culture systems (Table 1.1) will significantly advance the opportunities in this area. The following chapters address all the new areas highlighted above and suggest new possibilities for taking low throughput toxicology *in vitro* into sensitive HTS for preclinical lead optimization.

2 Automation and Technology for HTS in Drug Development

M. Banks, Bristol-Meyers Squib, Wallingford, USA

2.1 Introduction

The search for new medicines is one of the central themes in a broad disciplinary approach to tackling human disease. This chapter will focus essentially on the technology that is being used in the high throughput screening approach to drug discovery.

A critical step in the search for new medicines is to identify a unique property of a diseased cell, usually at a molecular level. This knowledge is then used to find or design a molecule that is capable of exploiting this property while ignoring all other biochemical events in the body. This is by no means a trivial task, but, nevertheless, this approach has yielded many important new medicines.

Having defined a potential biological target, the next step is to identify a molecule which has the ability to modulate that target in a desired fashion. High throughput screening is one method for finding this molecule. As the name implies, this involves taking hundreds of thousands of different chemicals and testing them against a biological target. This testing, in screening assays, is usually carried out using a range of biological systems, e.g. biochemical assays and cell-based assays. It is beyond the scope of this chapter to describe these screening assay types in detail and the interested reader is directed to an article by Wallace and Goldman (1997).

2.2 High throughput screening

High throughput screening (HTS) is more than a series of repetitive tests; it involves an entire cyclical process including chemistry, biology, engineering and informatics. A

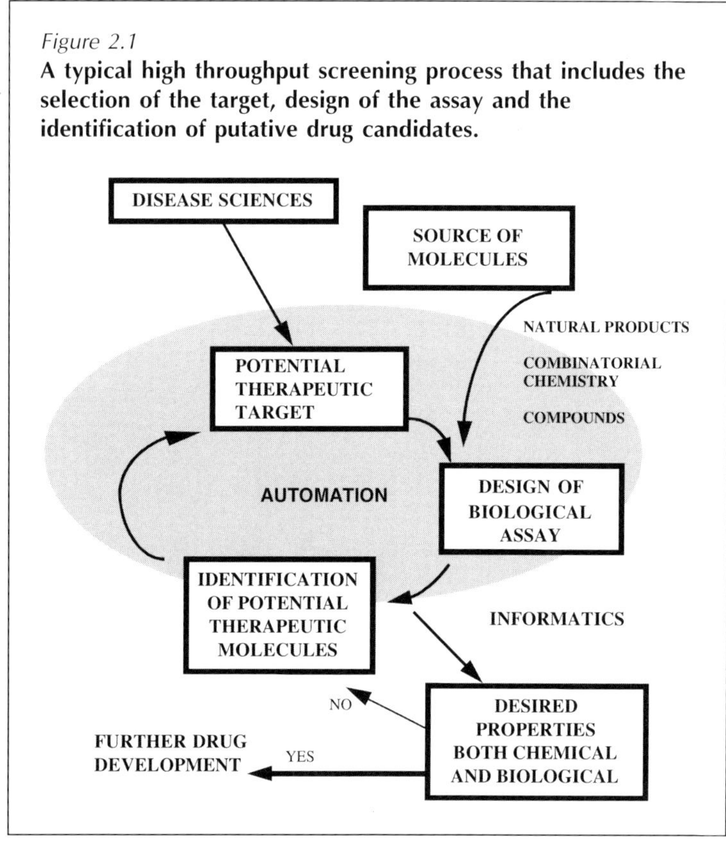

Figure 2.1

A typical high throughput screening process that includes the selection of the target, design of the assay and the identification of putative drug candidates.

typical HTS process is shown in Figure 2.1. Critical to the success of this process is the source of chemicals made available for screening against the biological target. Natural products that include plant extracts, both terrestrial and marine, and microbial fermentation products have been a rich source of structurally diverse chemical species for many decades. Some of the world's best known medicines have their origin in natural product chemistry. Examples include digitalis for cardiovascular disease, cyclosporin for preventing transplant rejection, and cephalosporins for bacterial infections, to name but a few. These sources remain an important feedstock of molecules for high throughput screening. Another popular source is proprietary pharmaceutical company compound collections that have been procured over many decades. These have usually been supplemented by a variety of chemicals that have been obtained commercially, either from specialist companies or from academic laboratories. Finally, an increasingly important source of new chemical entities is being provided by combinatorial chemistry. Traditional medicinal chemistry involved taking a

Figure 2.2

An example of a 'Split-Pool' approach to combinatorial chemistry. This scheme shows the addition of two functional groups, *A* and *C*, to a common core group *B* using solid phase synthesis on beads.

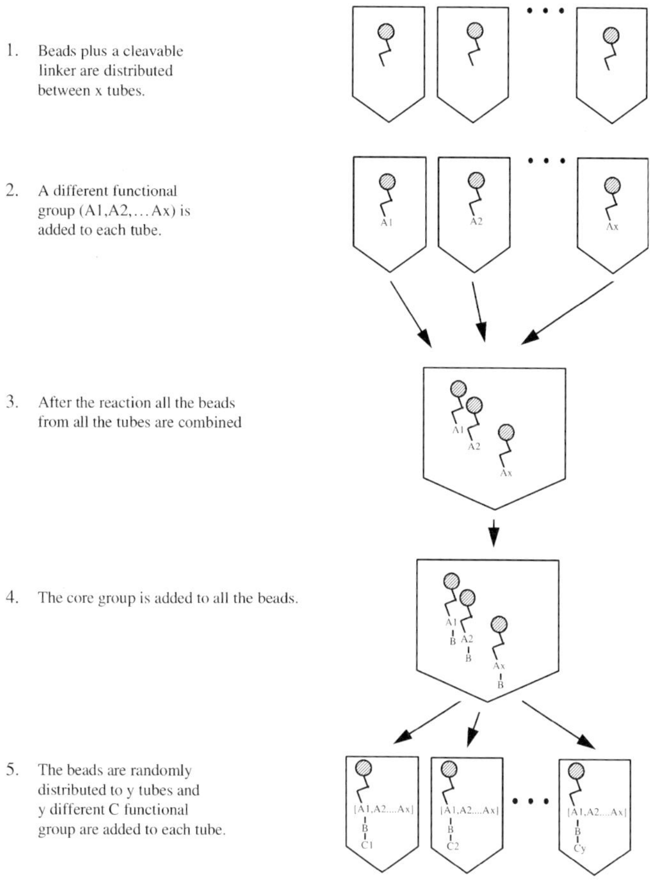

single molecule, modifying it and supplying it for biological evaluation. Based on the biological result this procedure was repeated in a serial manner until a molecule with the desired features was obtained. Combinatorial chemistry allows parallelization of this process so that the chemical space within a molecular series can be explored simultaneously. Usually these libraries are prepared using either solid phase support resins or as solution phase libraries.

A typical solid phase 'Split-Pool' (Houghton, 1985) combinatorial chemistry scheme is described in Figure 2.2. In this example A and C depict a range of monomers that are attached to a common central scaffold, B. If we consider the scheme described in Figure 2.2, at the end of the chemical synthesis there would be Y pools of X compounds in each tube. If a particular pool is found to be positive, this identifies the *C* functional group. The library can then be re-prepared, fixing both *B* and *C* such that the identity of *A* can be determined.

A whole variety of innovative systems are now available for preparing and screening combinatorial libraries (Gordon *et al.*, 1994; Wilson and Czarnik, 1997) and many of the syntheses are fully automated (Cargill *et al.*, 1995).

With increasing numbers of compounds becoming available for HTS, there is a need to design a process to introduce these compounds to the biological assay. To make this an efficient process one has to consider the physical state of the compounds. Ideally, all the compounds are stored as dry powders under an inert atmosphere in the dark and at low temperature. Therefore, an automated system would involve an electronic inventory, a standard compound bottle and racks that can be moved by a robotic arm. The robotic arm would deliver the rack or individual storage bottle to a weighing station. Here, a specified quantity would be removed and provided to the biologists for pharmacological assessment. Supervisory software would instruct the robot to return the compound storage bottle and update the inventory. Most proprietary compound storage systems have evolved over many years and consequently a whole range of storage jars has been used. Therefore a significant amount of effort is required to standardize the store. Furthermore, not all compounds are free flowing dry powders: a reasonable proportion of compounds exists as heterogeneous particle sizes, oils or other viscous liquids. These types of compounds invariably require manual dispensing, as automated machines capable with dealing with all these physical states are currently unavailable. Typically, the system described above will dispense 0.5–1 mg with accuracy and precision. As HTS assays only use micrograms of compound there is potential for considerable waste unless the compound is screened in multiple biological assays. Secondly, a HTS will assay anywhere between 10^5–10^6 compounds in a few weeks and this throughput can not be matched by the current designs of automated dry compound stores.

To overcome this bottleneck in the process a range of different pharmaceutical and biotechnological companies have invested in compound liquid stores. Generally there are two types of liquid store using tubes or deep well microtitre plates. Both these types of repositories take dry compounds dissolved in a suitable solvent, usually dimethyl sulphoxide, and store them for a limited time. In the tube based system individual compounds are stored in individual tubes. On request, the automated system retrieves these individual tubes and puts them into convenient blocks, usually based on a 96-well microtitre plate footprint. These compounds are then sent either directly for biological assay or to a 96-head pipetting device that removes an aliquot from each tube before returning them to the store. The obvious efficiency saving here is that it eliminates the need for repeated compound weighing, however, this type of system is still too slow to feed a typical HTS. An alternative automation solution is to store the soluble compounds in microtitre plates. When a request is made an entire plate, up to 96 compounds are retrieved at once. The disadvantage is that if only one compound is required from that block, there is potential for waste. However, one would normally store compounds in blocks based either on chemical class or known biological activity and also a typical HTS would not be requesting individual compounds. Having screened the compounds supplied by the plate liquid store, individual compounds of interest can now be requested from the tube based liquid store or from the dry compound store for further study.

2.3   Automation of the biological assay

Until recently HTS has been conducted exclusively using the 96-well microtitre plate as the assay format. Plates with 96 wells are widely available from many manufacturers and distributors, and come in a broad range of well shapes, materials, colours and surface treatments, designed to cater for the very wide variety of applications in the life sciences industry. Some manufacturers even describe themselves as 'microtitre plate boutiques', specializing in providing small quantities of custom designs of plates for specific esoteric applications.

In spite of its widespread use, there is no 'industry standard' 96-well plate: all manufacturers produce different designs with slightly different dimensions. These variations are usually unimportant where plates are being handled by human operators, however, the requirements of robotic handling systems dictate a need for tighter tolerances and increased standardization between plate manufacturers. The screening community (Astle, 1996) is now addressing this issue.

A typical high throughput screen will consist of processing hundreds, or even thousands, of 96-well microtitre plates

A typical high throughput screen will consist of processing hundreds, or even thousands, of 96-well microtitre plates through all the steps of an assay.

through all the steps of an assay. To support the use of the microtitre plate in screening, a wide range of instruments and devices is commercially available, to perform liquid-handling, incubation, washing, centrifugation, sealing, and detection.

Liquid-handling instruments in regular use range from entirely manually-operated pipetting devices, single or multi-channel, through to fully automated robotic sample processors, which can be used in stand-alone mode on a benchtop, or can be integrated into robotic systems as described elsewhere in this chapter. All the conventional devices are based on either some form of syringe-pump technology to provide volumetric precision, or on multi-channel peristaltic pumps that offer higher speed at the expense of some precision.

Many reading instruments are available specifically for use with microtitre plates. The conventional instruments are broadly based upon light emission/detection techniques: prompt fluorescence, optical density, luminescence, scintillation events and fluorescence polarization, are typical. Emission is generally achieved with a xenon flash source or laser source; detection is performed by one or more photomultiplier tubes, which may be cooled to reduce noise, or by a solid-state CCD chip camera, which might also be cooled to reduce noise. Some detectors are highly sophisticated and include built-in 96-channel liquid dispensers to add an assay component while simultaneously illuminating and imaging the entire plate, thereby allowing the study of rapid kinetic processes in 96 wells in parallel (Schroeder and Neagle, 1996).

For any biological assay, all of the operations that need to be performed can be clearly defined. Taking a range of assays, similar operations become evident. These have been termed 'Laboratory Unit Operations', LUO, which can be used to define the operational envelope of an automated system. As automated systems have become more popular, biological assay technology has evolved to become more amenable to automation; e.g. scintillation proximity assay (Cook, 1996). Scintillation proximity assay is ideally suited to automation because the assay is homogeneous; i.e. reagents are added to a microtitre plate and, after a suitable incubation period, a measurement is made. There is no need to remove the material from the reaction well for further processing. The principle of the technique is based on a plastic bead that contains a fluor and an outer hydrophilic coating to which biological molecules can be attached. Where a receptor has been attached to a bead a [³H] ligand can be measured in the presence of free ligand. While the ligand is bound to the receptor the tritium is in close proximity to the bead and on decay the beta particle will excite the fluor. A beta particle from a ligand in free solution will yield its energy to the surrounding medium before encountering a bead. Therefore, only bound tritium will cause light emission. For this type of assay the only LUOs required for scintillation proximity assays are racking to hold microtitre plates, liquid handling and scintillation counting (Mellor *et al.*, 1997).

Certain devices have been built which perform an automated function or with which a single or limited group of LUOs are performed. These workstations range from the very simple, e.g. a microtitre plate colorimeter, to the more complex liquid handling machines, like the Biomek 2000™ or Tecan Genesis™. Both these workstations perform Cartesian movement in the x, y, and z axes. Microtitre plates and reagent reservoirs are precisely located on a deck and a pipetting device moves liquids from reservoir to plate, and from plate to plate. An alternative approach is to place microtitre plates in stackers that feed plates to a fixed pipetting head then out to a second stacker, e.g. Matrix PlateMate™ or Multidrop™.

Integrated automation systems go one stage further and link all the workstations via a robotic arm. These robotic arms can be moved along a rail or stay static where they work with a predefined circle. Companies such as Zymark™ have used this circular robot approach where they have divided this working envelope into a series of sections, so-called Py-Sections™. The LUOs required are then assigned to a Py-Section. To increase the number of LUOs a considerable number of companies now produce robots that move on tracks or rail systems. The main advantage of the rail is that larger systems can be put together.

The next step in the evolution of automated high throughput screening system is the fully integrated turnkey system (Banks *et al.*, 1997). All the LUOs are functionally linked together by the robot arm under the control of supervisory software. Collectively these components are capable of performing a complete bioassay starting with a compound microtitre plate to data being sent to a corporate database. Human operators are responsible for loading microtitre plates onto the system, supplying or replenishing reagents and removing any waste. To build such a system there needs to be considerable financial investment and management commitment to support such a programme. A case history of the procurement of such a system has been described in detail elsewhere (Harding *et al.*, 1997).

Assays are designed to run these integrated systems, however certain assay types present considerable technical difficulties; e.g. a critical instrument may not be currently available in a configuration compatible with robot operation. Fully integrated systems do offer the following advantages:

a) Continuous operation

A stable system will run continuously overnight and through weekends, with only brief visits being necessary to renew reagents, remove waste and perform quality control checks. A proper workplan needs to be incorporated into the screening operation to include both hardware and biological assay quality control to achieve continuous operation.

b) Consistency of process

Every microtitre plate is treated exactly the same and interrogation of the system software allows verification of the entire process. This consistency allows precise planning of the entire screening operation so that everything from the supply of raw materials to the biological data output can be guaranteed.

c) Automated data tracking

The use of barcodes eliminates any errors in associating samples with biological assay data. This allows a particular result to be tracked right back to the compound store.

d) Safety

Our integrated screening systems are totally enclosed and interlocked which, together with waste management systems, dramatically reduces human exposure to potential hazards and minimizes environmental impact. For example, in a radiochemical assay the operator prepares reagents once a day and loads the robot. At any one time, only a relatively small number of plates are in process, minimizing exposure to isotope. Again, as biological materials and compounds are confined, human exposure is minimized.

e) Reduced operator boredom

The modern homogeneous screening procedures are tedious to perform manually or in a semi-automated mode. In these later screening processes the human operator is reduced to an automaton processing microtitre plates in monotonous manner. Automated systems require less operator attention.

A more detailed debate concerning the advantages and disadvantages of total integrated systems versus workstations have been discussed elsewhere.

2.4 Miniaturization trends in high throughput screening

2.4.1 Drivers for miniaturization of HTS

The main drivers for the miniaturization of high throughput screening are set out below. These drivers have different weight depending on the particular application: companies specializing in rapid screening of large numbers of liquid samples are driven largely by the cost savings per unit of throughput, whilst those specializing in the screening of bead-based libraries are driven rather by the need to increase concentrations.

2.4.2 Cost savings per unit of throughput

> Miniaturization allows the cost of processing a given number of samples to be driven down.

Miniaturization allows the cost of processing a given number of samples to be driven down. These savings, which arise from a number of factors, could be seen as an opportunity to reduce budgets while maintaining throughput, but in practice it is likely that most large pharmaceutical companies will instead use miniaturization to increase throughput while maintaining budgets. This is because the development of combinatorial chemistry and human genomics is leading to massive increases in the number of samples to be screened and the number of targets to screen against. This inevitably creates continual pressure to increase throughputs.

> The development of combinatorial chemistry and human genomics is leading to massive increases in the number of samples to be screened and the number of targets to screen against.

Labware savings. Miniaturization to higher density formats produces obvious savings by reducing the number of plates that must be bought to process a given number of samples. A regular microtitre plate costs typically £1–2; microtitre plate manufacturers currently charge a premium for high-density plates, but it is hoped that this will diminish over time as development and tooling charges are amortized and increased supply competition develops.

Reagent savings. A typical high throughput screening assay in 96-well microtitre plates will use a total assay volume of between 100 µl and 200 µl; reagent costs might typically be of the order of £10 per plate. These reagents might for example be specifically engineered proteins or radiolabelled ligand. Clearly, by reducing the assay volume to around 10 µl, major cost savings can be achieved.

Sample savings. The samples that are used in high throughput screening might be synthesized compounds, produced either by individual discrete synthesis or by combinatorial synthesis, or they might be natural product extracts. In either case they are a finite resource: miniaturization allows the samples to go further. It is difficult to quantify the savings this produces.

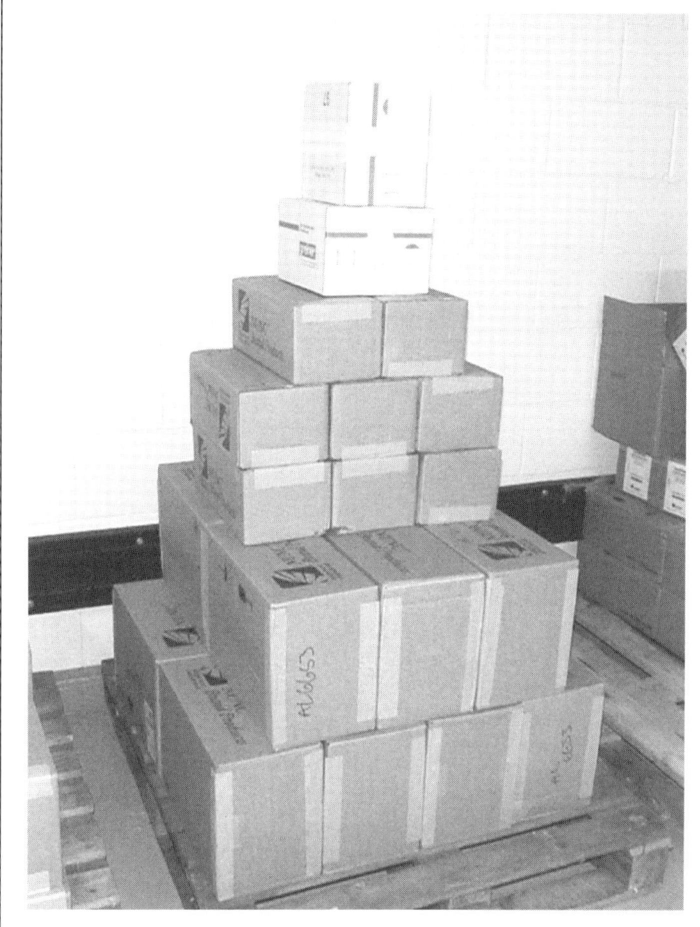

Figure 2.3a
A typical HTS screen campaign (c 200k datapoints): the lower group of fourteen 96-plate boxes (2000 plates) will typically require 1–2 months to screen. By contrast the middle group of six 384-plates (500 plates) can be screened in 1–2 weeks, while the two boxes of 1536 plates (125 plates) may be screened in 1–2 days. Picture courtesy of John Comley, Glaxo Wellcome.

Logistics savings. A conventional high throughput screening laboratory, based around the 96-well microtitre plate, requires a major logistical infrastructure to support it. Every high throughput screen requires the movement of large numbers of plates, tens of thousands per annum for one screening robot. Managing the ordering and QC checking of reagents, the disposal of solid and liquid waste, the supply of samples, the ongoing technological support for the auto-mation system, and many other ancillary processes, is not

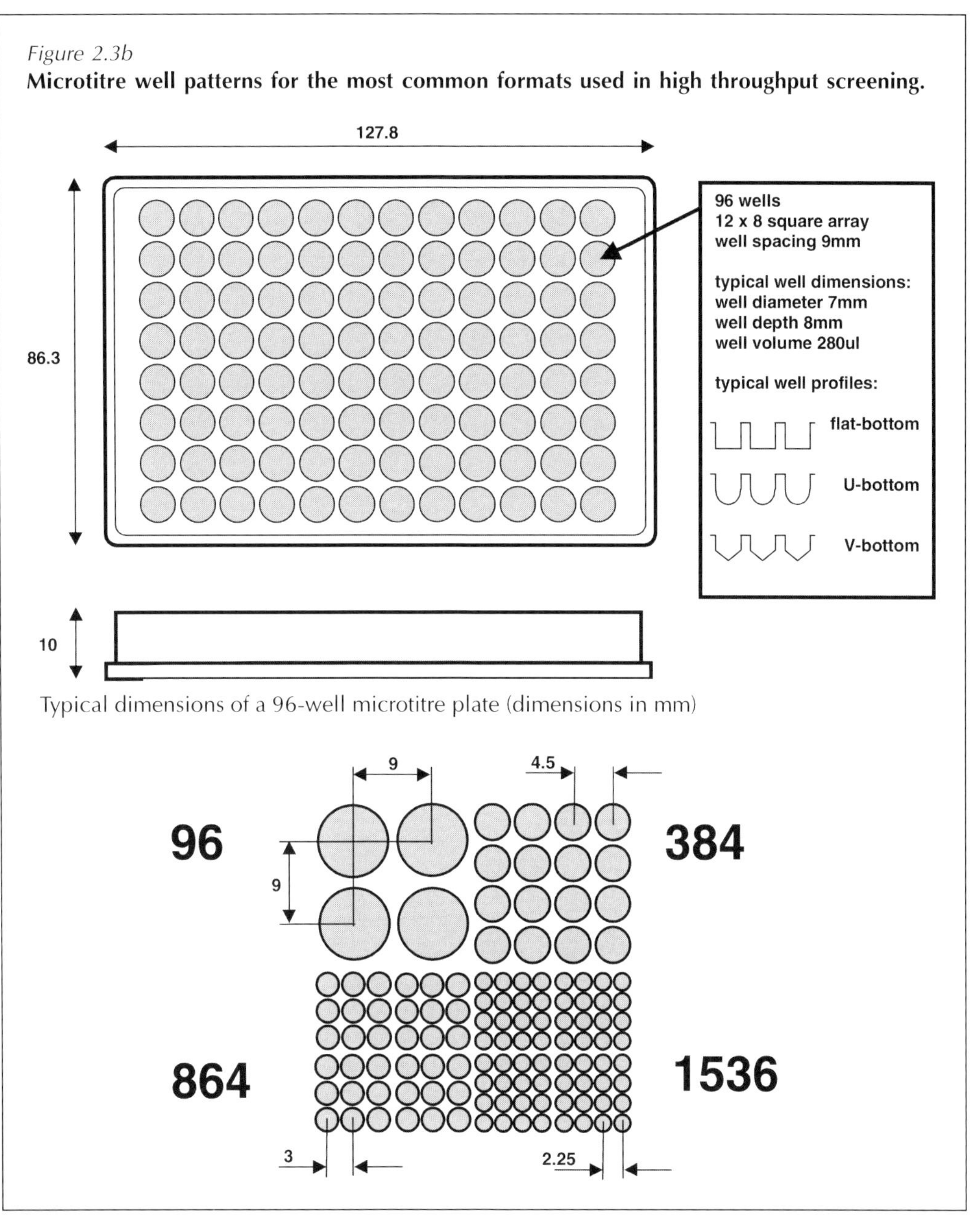

an insignificant task. The efficient orchestration of all this requires specialist staff, careful planning, and a very high degree of organization. It is difficult to quantify these costs but it is reasonable to surmise that the logistic costs correlate broadly with the number of plates that must be transferred around the operation. Figures 2.3a and 2.3b illustrate how the number of plates required for a current screening run is reduced to manageable proportions by miniaturization to 1536.

2.4.3 Increased concentrations from bead-based libraries

A further driver for miniaturization, entirely independent of cost savings, arises from current developments in combinatorial chemistry, where compounds are synthesized using macroporous polystyrene beads as a solid support. The beads are typically 100 μm to 300 μm in diameter. A single bead might yield a maximum 100 pmoles of compound for assaying, so in a 96-well microtitre plate with an assay volume of 200 μl, this results in a compound concentration in the screen of 0.5 μM. It is desirable to increase this concentration by at least one order of magnitude to allow the detection of less active compounds. A number of the prominent combinatorial chemistry companies are actively developing miniaturized screening systems for this reason.

> In combinatorial chemistry, compounds are synthesized using macroporous polystyrene beads as a solid support.

2.4.4 Use of precious reagents/primary cells

Currently, primary cells are never used in high throughput screening, and some reagents cannot be considered because of their prohibitive cost or short shelf life. Miniaturization potentially allows a much wider range of cells and reagents to be applied in high throughput.

> Miniaturization potentially allows a much wider range of cells and reagents to be applied in high throughput.

2.4.5 High-density microtitre plates

Beyond the 96-well plate, a number of higher-density formats are now emerging. All use the same nominal 128 mm × 86 mm footprint, with minor dimensional variations as seen with 96-well plates. Figures 2.4a and 2.4b illustrate some of the variations.

2.4.6 Issues in changing to higher-density formats

In deciding which of these formats to adopt, a high throughput screening operation has to consider the following issues:

There must be a sufficient range of plates available in the new format. Typically, to support the range of assay types and storage requirements, one might require assay plates to be clear (for OD reading), black (for fluorescence reading), white (for luminescence or scintillation applications), white or black with transparent well bases (for reading fluorescence or luminescence/scintillation from below without cross-talk).

Typical 96-well plates used for sample storage and high throughput screening.

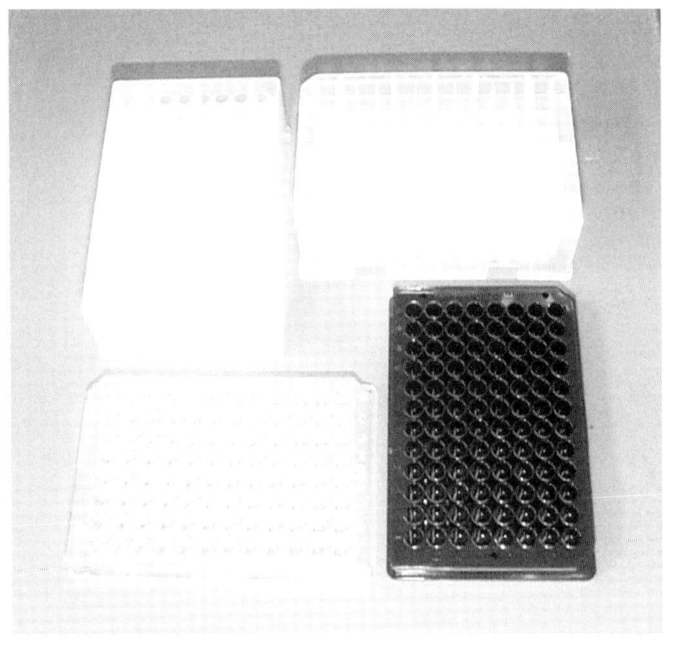

High-density microtitre plates. Clockwise from lower right: 1536 square wells (Greiner); 384 round wells (Genetix); 384 square wells (Nunc); 864 round wells (Helix).

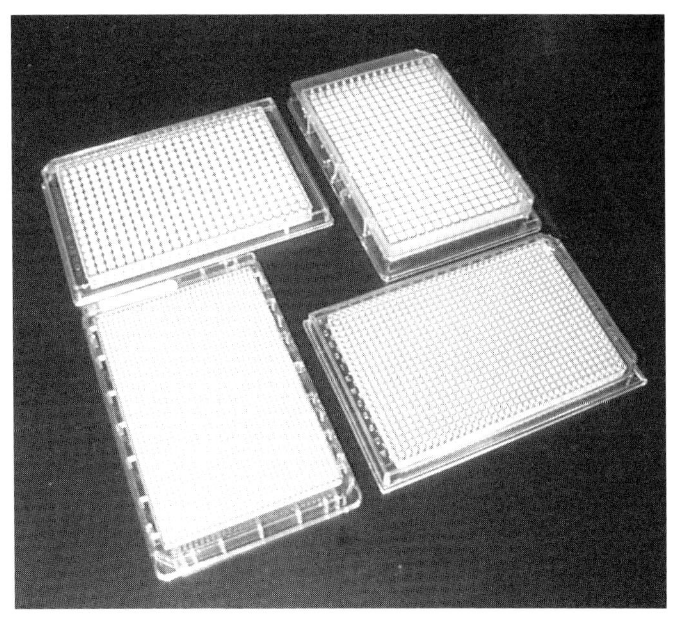

These are normally injection-molded in a variety of grades of polystyrene, with a range of fillers to provide the appropriate optical properties. Tissue culture treated plates might be required for cell-based assays. One might also require higher volume plates for liquid sample storage, possibly in polypropylene because of its long-term inertness to storage solvents such as DMSO.

A sufficient range of bioassay types must run successfully in the volume allowed by the new format. This is likely to be particularly important for cell-based assays requiring uniform culture conditions within a well and/or long incubation periods without significant evaporation. It is also an issue in radiometric assays where very small volumes reduce the count rate towards background levels.

Introduction of a new format requires much upheaval of the operation's infrastructure; therefore the new format must offer a worthwhile improvement in costs or throughputs. As previously described, a high throughput screening operation is a large logistical effort and changing the basic unit of transfer could lead to major implications for people management, data-handling and bioinformatics infrastructure, materials and resource planning, and many other ramifications. While these changes are being implemented, productivity is inevitably reduced. Consequently, the change of format must offer a significant benefit to make this upheaval worthwhile.

2.4.7 *High-density microtitre plates currently available*

The 384-well plate is now being used more and more routinely in high throughput screening applications.

384. The 384-well plate is now being used more and more routinely in high throughput screening applications. It is now likely that over the next few years this format will supersede the 96-well plate as the industry standard for many assay types. This is because experience shows that a wide range of assays can be performed in 384-well plates using the instrumentation currently in routine use for 96-well plates. A typical 384-well plate offers assay volumes of up to 70 µl. The minimum practical assay volume is defined by liquid-handling restrictions and by the need to ensure that the bottom of the well is completely and evenly filled by the assay mixture to avoid meniscus effects distorting the signal reading. In practice 20 µl is a workable minimum assay volume (Janzen and Domanico, 1996; Kolb and Neumann, 1997).

Beyond the 384-well plate, a number of higher densities are now under development:

768. A leading US manufacturer has proposed a 768-plate (768 = 2 × 384) that allows direct transfers from 384-well plates using a 384-channel liquid dispenser.

864. An 864-well plate is available with approximately 2 mm diameter round wells and a depth of approximately 7 mm, yielding an assay volume of 20 μl. This plate was originally designed for high throughput PCR applications. The aspect ratio of wells of this design, which are very long and narrow compared to 96-well plates, makes them difficult to fill effectively. Liquid tends to cling to the side of the walls rather than drain to the bottom of the wells, so that the plates may require a centrifugation stage after each liquid addition, which severely detracts from their utility in a high throughput screening context (Comley *et al.*, 1997). A leading US combinatorial chemistry company has developed its own proprietary square-well 864-plate which has a much larger cross-sectional area per well and hence superior liquid-handling properties. This plate has been developed specifically for bead-based screening applications.

1536. Now that the high throughput screening industry is increasingly adopting the 384-well plate as the next standard after the 96-well plate, there is a developing view that the 864-well plate does not offer a sufficient advantage over 384 to make the transition worthwhile. Moving from 384 to 864 yields a cost/throughput ratio improvement factor of 2.25, and a similar reduction in the minimum practical volume. Consequently, there is an increasing consensus in the industry in favour of 1536 as the next standard beyond 384. A range of 1536 plates is available (Greiner GmbH, Frickenhausen, Germany) whose square wells (side c. 1.8 mm, depth c. 4 mm) give a working volume of c. 12 μl. A further range is available with working volume 1 μl (Corning Costar Corporation, Cambridge, Massachusetts, USA). In practice the larger volume plates are arguably of more utility at present, because of dispense limitations with current liquid-handling equipment and because of the very high rate of evaporation from the 1 μl plate. It has been shown that fluorescence and optical density can be read in 1536-well plates without a significant loss in signal strength or signal-to-noise ratio. Other manufacturers are currently in the process of developing their own versions of the 1536-well plate.

3456. A prototype 3456-well plate (3456 = 6^2 × 96) was developed at Glaxo (Norton, 1995) in 1994 at a time when the 96-well plate was the only format in use in high throughput screening. The wells on this 3456-well plate were of inverse square-pyramid shape and offered a working volume of

> There is an increasing consensus in the industry in favour of 1536 as the next standard beyond 384.

c. 0.5 µl. Due to the difficulties of solving all of the liquid-handling, bioassay development and detection challenges simultaneously, this development was abandoned in favour of a gradual progression from the 96-well plate to the 384-well plate and then beyond. More recently, Aurora Biosciences (Shumate, 1998) have proposed a high throughput screening system based on the use of 3456-well plates, known as 'nanoplates'.

9600. The highest plate density which is currently being actively worked upon is the 9600-well plate being developed at Merck Dupont (Oldenburg *et al.*, 1998). This has inverse square-pyramid wells with a working volume of 0.2 µl. The plate is injection-molded in liquid-crystal polymer and is still at an experimental stage, but in combination with inkjet-based dispensing technology and novel imaging detection techniques offers exciting possibilities for the future.

2.4.8 *Liquid-handling instruments for miniaturized assays*

In implementing a miniaturized HTS infrastructure using, for example, 1536 plates, probably the most critical technology challenges are in the area of liquid handling. For a generalized assay process, the liquid-handling tasks fall into four categories:

1. Sample reformatting: multi-channel re-formatting of entire plates (96 or 384) to create daughter 1536 plates, which can then be used as a 1536 store. A typical transfer volume would be 10 µl, which could then be used to supply 10–100 daughter screening plates.
2. Sample replication: creation of 1536 screening plates from 1536 store plates. Typical volume range will be 0.5 µl down to 50 nl. In this process it is often essential to minimize the volume transferred in order to minimize the concentration of sample carrier solvent in the final assay.
3. Cherry-picking of single samples from 1536 store plates to 1536 screen plates, to create retest plates, used to confirm activity from a primary screen, or dilution series, used to generate dose response data. The ideal volume range for this process in a 1536 system is from 1 µl down to 1 nl.
4. Bulk reagent dispensing of a common reagent from a reservoir to all wells of a 1536 plate (or to control wells only). Up to four common reagents may be required per assay. This may also include suspensions of viable cells. Typically the volume range will be 0.5–10 µl.

Figure 2.5
Liquid-handling instruments used for miniaturized HTS.

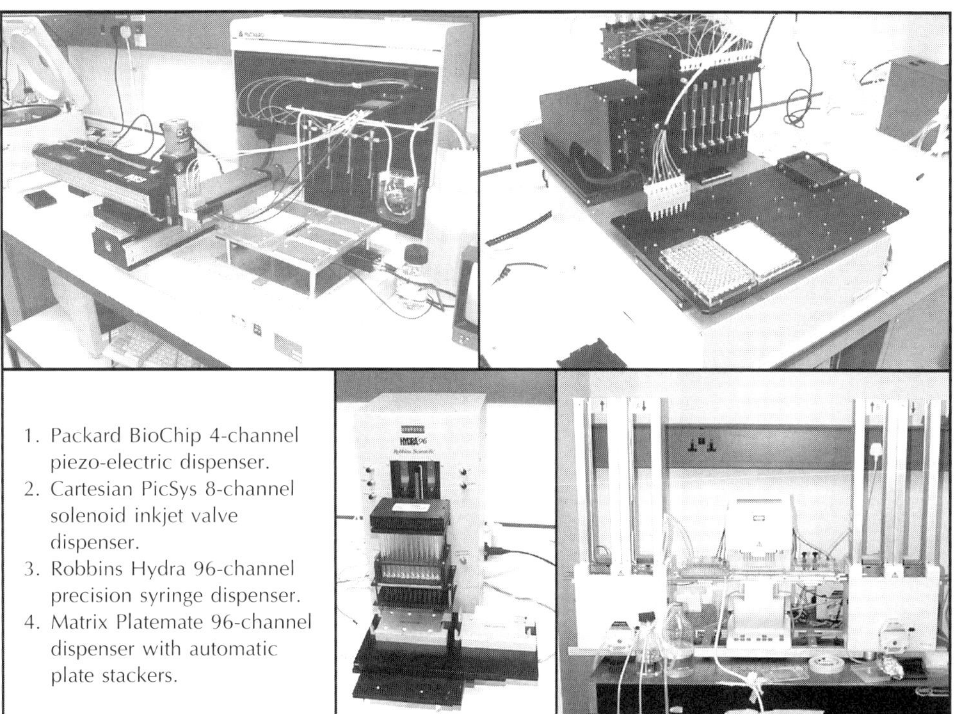

1. Packard BioChip 4-channel piezo-electric dispenser.
2. Cartesian PicSys 8-channel solenoid inkjet valve dispenser.
3. Robbins Hydra 96-channel precision syringe dispenser.
4. Matrix Platemate 96-channel dispenser with automatic plate stackers.

Typical instruments that can be used for these tasks are shown in Figure 2.5 [20–23]

- Matrix Platemate 96-channel dispenser (supplied by Matrix Technologies Corp., Lowell, MA, USA) with stackers and stage specially configured for 1536. This uses disposable tips, but also offers an on-line wash bath so that the tips may be re-used, which makes it ideal for sample transfers. The minimum transfer volume is 0.5 µl. This instrument is most useful for sample reformatting and reagent addition.
- Robbins Hydra 96-channel dispenser (supplied by Robbins Scientific, Sunnyvale, CA, USA) with automated stage, suitable for lower volumes than the Platemate. This instrument uses fixed steel capillary tips and precisely-made glass syringes, which provide superior low-volume precision. As such the instrument is suitable for sample reformatting, sample replication, and reagent addition. The absence of any plate-stacking facility means

that the use of this instrument for high throughput work is very labour-intensive.

- BioDot PicSys 8-channel solenoid inkjet dispenser (supplied by BioDot Ltd, Diddington, Cambs, UK). Each channel of this instrument uses a conventional precision syringe pump, with the additional feature that at the dispensing tip there is a miniature solenoid valve, based on the type used in continuous stream inkjet printing. This valve is driven synchronously with the steps of the syringe pump so as to act as a very precise metering valve. In this way the instrument can dispense (or aspirate) very low volumes. Minimum dispense volumes are about 10 nl. An additional advantage is that dispensing is non-contact: the pressure from the syringe pumps ensures that droplets are dynamically ejected from the dispenser tip. This means that the dispense precision is less affected by variations in target plate geometry and surface properties. The main application for this device is likely to be very rapid dispensing of common reagents; the limited number of channels restricts its applications for sample transfer.

- Packard BioChip 4-channel piezo-electric inkjet dispenser (supplied by Packard Biosciences, Meriden, CT, USA). Each channel of this instrument uses a conventional precision syringe pump, with the additional feature that at the dispensing tip there is a miniature piezo-electric valve. The syringe pump is used to aspirate and dispense in the normal way, and the piezo-electric valve is used as a metering valve to dispense very low-volume (c. 300 picolitres) droplets. Like the PicSys, this is a non-contact dispenser offering the advantage that the dispense precision is less affected by variations in target plate geometry and surface properties. The very low droplet volume allows an entire dilution series curve to be created using direct dispensing from a single aspirate. This instrument also has very precise spatial drives, making it ideal for cherry-picking individual samples from 1536 storage plates.

2.4.9 *Revolutionary approaches to miniaturization*

In discussing attempts to miniaturize high throughput screening, we have so far addressed what is essentially an 'evolutionary' strategy, in which the 96-well plate is gradually superseded by the 384-well plate, and then by a further short step the next higher density (e.g. 1536) is slowly introduced. Arguably, however, this makes no fundamental changes to the screening process: the logical conclusion of this approach is high throughput screening in microtitre plates with discrete wells, just at a higher density. This has the advantages of requiring only incremental innovations and gradual infrastructure re-engineering, so it represents a practical and relatively low-risk approach. As such it is likely that this is the strategy which will predominate in the industry for the next few years.

However, a more radical approach now being proposed by a number of companies and academic groups (Hook, 1996; Whitesides, 1997) is to apply the techniques of microfabrication to develop systems for high throughput screening which entirely abandon the conventional microtitre plate approach.

Microfabrication techniques originated in the microelectronics industry, but recently it has been shown extensively that, in addition to solid-state electronic devices, the same basic techniques can be used to fabricate a wide range of sensors, actuators and fluidics devices. It is therefore possible to design devices which combine fluid channels, pumps and valves, mechanisms, electro-optics, biosensors or chemosensors, specially-textured surfaces to encourage and direct cell growth, with conventional electronic devices to create the so-called 'lab-on-a-chip'. These might ultimately allow assays to be performed at nanolitre volumes. A number of such devices have been reported (Kopf-Sill, 1998; Conway, 1997) and this is a rapidly expanding and very exciting multi-disciplinary field.

However, most of the currently published devices are for well-defined and quite specific applications, and have been developed in an academic context. They do not offer the generality and robustness that would be required in high throughput screening. The challenge now is to develop devices which can be configured for a range of assay types and which will be sufficiently cheap, robust and stable to use in an industrial context.

2.5   Conclusions

The high throughput screening industry is currently in a state of transition, being driven to miniaturization by the need to increase throughput but decrease costs. Over the next few years, developments in bioware technology, liquid-handling techniques and imaging will enable the adoption of the 1536 plate for many applications. However, the instrumentation is likely to be expensive and, in some cases, specialized so it is likely that the 96-well plate will also

'Lab-on-a-chip' technology will advance to the point where it is possible to operate an entire high throughput sample supply and screening operation from a small, highly-integrated benchtop workstation.

remain with us for some applications for the foreseeable future. In the long-term future, it may be envisaged that 'lab-on-a-chip' technology will advance to the point where it is possible to operate an entire high throughput sample supply and screening operation (which currently requires large and specialist capital equipment in dedicated laboratories) from a small, highly-integrated benchtop workstation.

References

Astle, T., 1996, Report from the Committee on Microplate Standardization for Automated Handling, *J. Biomolecular Screening*, **1**, 163–168.

Banks, M., Binnie, A. and Fogarty, S.J., 1997, High throughput screening using fully integrated robotic screening, *J. Biomolecular Screening*, **2**, 133–135.

Cargill, J.F., Maiefski, R.R. and Toyonaga, B.E., 1995, Automated combinatorial chemistry on solid phase, *Proc. Int. Symp. Lab. Autom. Robotics*, 221–234.

Comley, J.C.W., Binnie, A., Bonk, C. and Houston, J.G., 1997, A 384-HTS for human factor VIIa: comparison with 96- and 864-well formats, *J. Biomolecular Screening*, **2**, 171–178.

Conway, P., 1997, 'A massively-parallel, microfabricated system for synthesis and screening of small molecules', presentation at Drug Discovery Technology 97, San Diego, CA, USA.

Cook, N.D., 1996, Scintillation proximity assay – a versatile high throughput screening technology, *Drug Dis. Today*, **1**, 287–294.

Gordon, E.M., Barrett, R.W., Dower, W.J., Fodor, S.P.A. and Gallop, M., 1994, Applications of combinatorial technologies to drug discovery: 2. Combinatorial organic synthesis, library screening strategies and future directions, *J. Med. Chem.*, **37**, 1385–1401.

Harding, D., Banks, M., Fogarty, S. and Binnie, A., 1997, Development of an automated screening system: a case history, *Drug Dis. Today*, **2**, 385–390.

Hook, D., 1996, Ultra-high throughput screening – a journey into nanoland with Gulliver and Alice, *Drug Dis. Today*, **1**, 267–268.

Houghton, R.A., 1985, General method for the rapid solid-phase synthesis of large numbers of peptides: specificity of antigen–antibody interaction at the level of individual amino acids, *Proc. Natl. Acad. Sci. USA*, **82**, 5131–5135.

Janzen, B. and Domanico, P., 1996, The 384-well plate: pros and cons, *J. Biomolecular Screening*, **1**, 63–64.

Kolb, A.J. and Neumann, K., 1997, Beyond the 96-well microplate: instruments and assay methods for the 384-well format, *J. Biomolecular Screening*, **2**, 103–109.

Kopf-Sill, A., 1998, 'Lab-on-a-chip', presentation at Lab-Automation 1998, San Diego, CA, USA.

Mellor, G.W., Fogarty, S.J., O'Brien, M.S., Congreve, M., Banks, M.N., Mills, K.M. *et al.*, 1997, Searching for chemokine receptor binding antagonists by high throughput screening, *J. Biomolecular Screening*, **2**, 153–157.

Norton, D.W.J., 1995, A prototype 3456 plate for ultra-high throughput screening, unpublished personal communication.

Oldenburg, K.R. *et al.*, 1998, Assay miniaturization for ultra-high throughput screening of combinatorial and discrete compound libraries: a 9600 0.2 microlitre assay system, *J. Biomolecular Screening*, **3**, 55–62.

Schroeder, K.S. and Neagle, B.D., 1996, FlipR: A new instrument for rapid, optical high throughput screening, *J. Biomolecular Screening*, **1**, 75–80.

Shumate, C.B., 1998, 'Ultra-high throughput screening: industrializing the drug discovery process', presentation at LabAutomation 1998, San Diego, CA, USA.

Wallace, R.W. and Goldman, M.E., 1997, Bioassay design and implementation, in Devlin, J.P. (ed.), *High Throughput Screening: the Discovery of Bioactive Substances*, Marcel Decker, pp. 279–305.

Whitesides, G., 1997, 'Microtechnology and drug discovery', keynote address at Drug Technology 97, San Diego, CA, USA.

Wilson, S.R. and Czarnik, A.W. (eds), 1997, *Combinatorial Chemistry: Synthesis and Applications*, New York: Wiley Interscience.

3 Cytotoxicity and Mechanistic Studies in High Throughput Toxicity Screening

Jeffrey R. Fry, Queen's Medical Centre, Nottingham

3.1 Introduction

As outlined elsewhere in this book, recent advances in organic chemistry (combinatorial chemistry) and pharmacology (transfection of cells in culture to allow expression of specific molecular targets) have led to the development of large chemical libraries and their subsequent high throughput screening (HTS) for pharmacological activity. From this approach a limited number of acceptable 'hits' will be identified which possess the required pharmacological activity, and priorities will then need to be established to determine which compounds go further into lead development and the process of lead optimization. It is recognized that toxicity and an unfavourable pharmacokinetic profile are frequent reasons for failure of new chemical entities during drug development. It is, therefore, logical to set in place toxicity and pharmacokinetic screens to act as secondary filters in the lead optimization phase of development candidate selection, subsequent to the primary pharmacology HTS. In some cases, and indeed in some commercial organizations and therapeutic areas, however, it is not uncommon to find basal cytotoxicity screens (employing cell lines) operative alongside efficacy HTS.

At this point it is relevant to consider in more depth what is being hoped for in conducting a toxicity screen, and the differences between this and the pharmacology and pharmacokinetics screens. In the latter two screens, well-defined endpoints can be established which clearly indicate the approaches to pursue in the development of a valid screen. Thus in the pharmacology screen what needs to be measured is some expression of the interaction of a chemical with an identified cellular target, whereas in the pharmacokinetic screens the issues of concern are the absorption characteristics of the drug from an oral dose and its metabolic stability. The phenomenon of drug toxicity, on the other hand, comprises the possible involvement of any one of a number of target organs, mechanisms, and manifestations of functional or structural impairment. This situation is clearly different from those encountered in trying to establish pharmacological and pharmacokinetic profiles, and the challenge to *in vitro* toxicologists is the development and validation of sensible *in vitro* approaches for the generation of toxicity profiles in the context of HTS. This represents the theme of this chapter, and the following discussion is based on two premises – first, that it will not be possible to identify all mechanisms of toxicity in a toxicity screen, and, second, that a battery of tests/approaches will be required to generate a sensible toxicity profile.

With regard to the first premise, it should be realized that the exact combination of mechanism of toxicity and target organ/cell type could be unique to each chemical, so that emphasis should be given to identifying mechanisms of toxicity and target organs which are common to a large number of chemicals. By accepting this, efforts can be focused on devising *in vitro* screens to these common problems, while accepting that not all mechanisms/target organs can be screened.

With regard to the second premise, it is likely that input from a variety of sources – quantitative structure-activity relationships (QSAR), cytotoxicity data, mechanistic information, stress response, *etc.* – will give the most comprehensive information on the likely toxicity of a compound. This premise is attested to by the range of topics covered elsewhere in this book, particularly the chapters on QSAR and stress responses; for this reason, this chapter focuses on the role of cytotoxicity studies and mechanistic information in devising *in vitro* toxicology screens.

3.2 Basal cytotoxicity screens

Considerable effort has been expended over the last few years in devising *in vitro* culture-based systems for the assessment of xenobiotic toxicity, the driving force for this being the desire to predict acute toxicity. A number of useful reviews of this area have recently been published (Fry, 1993; Guzzie, 1994; Garle *et al.*, 1994; Seibert *et al.*, 1996).

> The exact combination of mechanism of toxicity and target organ/cell type could be unique to each chemical, so that emphasis should be given to identifying mechanisms of toxicity and target organs which are common to a large number of chemicals.

Basal cytotoxicity involves adverse effects on those structures/ functions which are common to all cell types.

Selective cytotoxicity represents cytotoxicity to a particular cell type as a consequence of some differentiated function.

Cell-specific function toxicity involves toxic effects on structures or processes which are critical to the organism as a whole.

The central premise of this approach, recently elaborated by Seibert *et al.* (1996), has been that chemicals can exert one (or more) of three types of toxic effect at the cellular level, and that all three types of effect can result in acute toxicity *in vivo. Basal cytotoxicity* involves adverse effects on those structures/functions which are common to all cell types (e.g. plasma membrane integrity, mitochondrial energy production, etc.), and which would be expected to be similar across a variety of cell systems. *Selective cytotoxicity* represents cytotoxicity to a particular cell type as a consequence of some differentiated function (e.g. biotransformation, receptor activation, etc.); this would obviously require testing in the appropriate differentiated cells to observe the effect. *Cell-specific function toxicity* involves toxic effects on structures or processes, which may not be critical for the affected cells themselves, but which are critical to the organism as a whole (e.g. cytokine, hormone or neurotransmitter release and actions). It is very unlikely that such toxicity could be modelled *in vitro* in a form suitable for HTS.

Basal cytotoxicity can be readily modelled *in vitro.* For example, the toxicity of anti-tumour compounds and metabolic inhibitors (which would be expected to cause toxicity by impairment of cell basal functions) to an undifferentiated cell line shows a significant positive correlation with acute toxicity *in vivo*, as measured by LD_{50} values (Fry *et al.*, 1990). Three other notable features emerged from this study. The first was that *in vitro* toxicity correlated better with i.p. or i.v. LD_{50} values than with oral LD_{50} values, as previously predicted (Fry *et al.*, 1988). This finding has also been reported elsewhere (Weiss and Sawyer, 1993). Secondly, the *in vivo – in vitro* correlations were much better for subsets of chemicals with identical modes of action (e.g. antimetabolites) than for the sample as a whole. Finally, marked deviations from the general pattern were apparent for those compounds which were either rapidly inactivated by metabolism or else metabolized to reactive metabolites, these deviations showing up as greater or lesser toxicity respectively *in vitro* relative to *in vivo.*

A wide variety of cell types, of both animal and human origin, and a wide variety of endpoints (cell number, cell protein, neutral red uptake, tetrazolium dye reduction, etc.) have been used in studies of basal cytotoxicity *in vitro.* However, the general consensus is that essentially identical results in terms of ranking chemical cytotoxicity are obtained irrespective of the choice of cell type or endpoint (Barile *et al.*, 1994; Garle *et al.*, 1994; Clemedson *et al.*, 1996; Järkelid *et al.*, 1997).

These considerations lead to a number of general conclusions on the use and interpretation of basal cytotoxicity tests as predictors of acute *in vivo* toxicity:

- The results obtained from these tests will provide a good estimate of the cell basal toxicity of a xenobiotic administered by the i.p. or i.v. route;
- The tests provide no information on the likelihood that basal cytotoxicity is the principal contributor to toxicity *in vivo*;
- Absorption from an oral dose may be a confounding variable (although an estimate of the extent of absorption may be obtained from the pharmacokinetic screen);
- Metabolism of the xenobiotic may also be a confounding variable.

In the context of HTS for toxicity, the most useful purpose in generating basal cytotoxicity data is to provide baseline data for other cell-based tests which probe for specific toxicity endpoints. This is likely to be true even if attempts are made to overcome the metabolism problem by using target cells that express some drug-metabolizing activity, as with rat or human (HepG2) hepatoma cells, because: a) the levels of drug-metabolizing capability in such cells is very low (see, for example, data for rat hepatoma cell line, Garle and Fry, 1996); and b) no attempt is made to identify metabolic activation as a mechanism of toxicity (see later).

3.3 Selective cytotoxicity

A number of well-characterized experimental *in vitro* systems are now available for studying selective cytotoxicity; examples in the areas of hepatotoxicity, neurotoxicity, reproductive toxicity, haematotoxicity, and nephrotoxicity, amongst others, may be found in various ECVAM (European Centre for the Validation of Alternative Methods) reports (Blaauboer *et al.*, 1994; Atterwill *et al.*, 1994; Brown *et al.*, 1995; Gribaldo *et al.*, 1996; Morin *et al.*, 1997). Such experimental systems have provided a wealth of information on mechanisms of toxicity, species differences, etc. which has then been used in many instances to aid in human risk assessment. However, it is becoming increasingly apparent that quite sophisticated culture techniques, such as organ spheroid culture, culture on extra-cellular matrix, use of particular growth factors, etc. are needed to model accurately the *in vivo* behaviour of most differentiated cells. In addition, most of the functionally-competent systems for selective

---

The most useful purpose in generating basal cytotoxicity data is to provide baseline data for other cell-based tests which probe for specific toxicity endpoints.

Sophisticated culture techniques are needed to model accurately the *in vivo* behaviour of most differentiated cells.

cytotoxicity are based on culture of animal or human material, rather than culture of continuous cell lines. Hence, use of these systems is dependent on the continued availability of fresh tissue, although considerable effort is being expended to establish functionally-competent immortalized cell lines to overcome this limitation. It is for these reasons (complex culture conditions, requirement for fresh tissue) that it is unlikely that cell-based tests for selective cytotoxicity would play a major role in HTS for toxicity, at least at the level of a secondary screen downstream of the pharmacology screen, although they will increasingly find application at the later stages of drug development, possibly as screens when a very truncated set of candidate drugs has been arrived at by continued rounds of screening.

3.4 Mechanistically-based tests for toxicity

An alternative approach that may be of benefit in the short- to medium-term takes a different starting point from the cell-based approaches, and is based on the premise that tests based upon a specific mechanism of toxicity will have useful predictive value if that mechanism is known to be common to a diverse set of chemicals.

One such 'common' mechanism of toxicity is that of metabolic activation to a reactive metabolite (Scheme A in Figure 3.1; Nelson and Pearson, 1990). Typically, a xenobiotic is metabolized by cytochrome P450 isoforms to a reactive metabolite which can either be inactivated by conjugation with the thiol-containing tripeptide glutathione (GSH) or bind to tissue protein via thiol residues and so initiate cellular damage. The archetype for this mechanism is the hepatotoxicity produced by large doses of paracetamol in humans. More recently, this paradigm has been refined to incorporate the existence of 'critical' and 'non-critical' protein targets, to account for the findings of covalent binding of reactive metabolite to protein in the absence of toxicity (Cohen *et al.*, 1997).

Various endpoints related to this mechanism have been used as measures of reactive metabolite generation *in vitro*, in particular: a) covalent binding of a radiolabelled substrate in the presence of tissue (usually liver) microsomes as a source of P450 and the appropriate cofactors for P450 function; and b) depletion of GSH in hepatocytes following exposure to the toxicant. Each of these approaches has disadvantages in the context of HTS – the requirement for radiolabelled substrate for a) and the reliance on fresh donor tissue for b).

Scheme B
Scheme A
Reductase
e⁻
Y
Y•
X
O₂
P450
O₂⁻•
[X]
OH•
H₂O₂
Conjugation
GSH
Oxidation
TOXICITY
GSH
Conjugate
H₂O
Covalent Binding
to Tissue Protein
via -SH Groups
TOXICITY

Figure 3.1

The central role of glutathione (GSH) as a cytoprotectant against xenobiotic toxicity mediated by covalent binding of reactive metabolite to tissue protein (Scheme A) and oxidative stress (Scheme B).

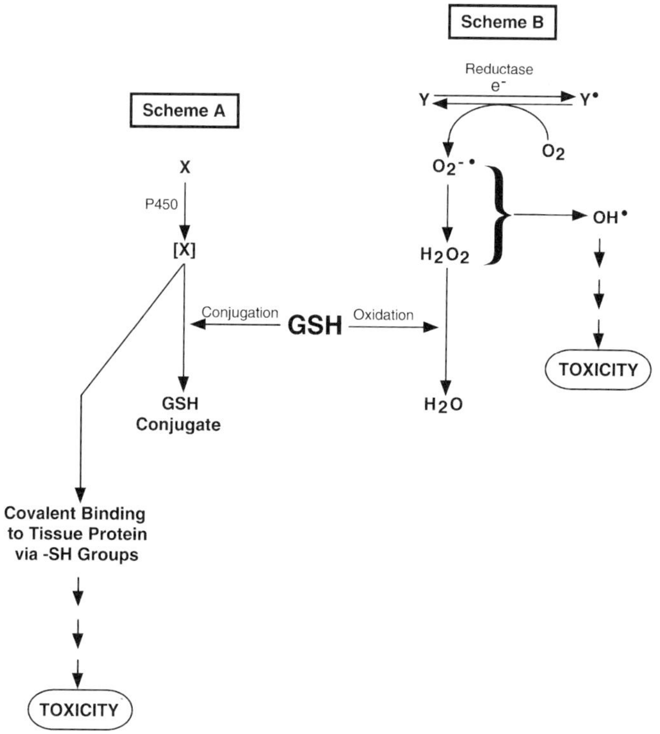

We have described a hybrid approach, based on the initial studies of Aikawa *et al.* (1978), which overcomes these disadvantages, and provides a reliable measure of the production of reactive metabolites which covalently bind to tissue protein via thiol residues (Garle and Fry, 1988). In this system, liver microsomes are incubated with substrate, cofactors, and added GSH, and the production of a reactive metabolite is detected by loss of this GSH. The chemicals that have produced a positive response in this assay to date are presented in Table 3.1; a positive response is taken to be ≥ 10% GSH depletion per milligram of microsomal protein over a 30-minute incubation time. A number of points can be made regarding these results and the assay in general:

1. All of these compounds (with the exception of 8-methoxycoumarin and 5,6-dihydro-2H-pyran-2-one for

Table 3.1 Diversity of xenobiotics which produce a positive response in the rat liver microsomal GSH depletion assay

Chemical	Microsome Dependence	Effect of P450 Induction
Allyl Alcohol	+	↑
Benzofuran (2,3-)	+	↑
Bromobenzene	+	↑
Bromophenol (4-)	+	↑
Butylated hydroxytoluene	+	↑
Chloroform	+	↑
Coumarin	+	↑
Cyclophosphamide	+	↑
Dichloro-2-propanol (1,3-)	+	↑
Dichloro-3-propanol (1,2-)	+	↑
Hydroxyacetanilide (3-)	+	↑
Ipomeanol (4-)	+	↑
Methoxsalen	+	↑
Methoxycoumarin (8-)	?	↑
Methylfuran (2-)	+	↑
Methylindole (3-)	+	↑
Morphine	+	↑
Paracetamol	+	↑
Precocene II	+	↑
Toluene	+	↑
Trichloroethylene	?	↑
Thiopurine	+	↓
Menadione	–/+	↑
Acrolein	–	↔ to ↑
Hexachlorobutadiene	–	↔ to ↑
Cyclohexen-1-one (2-)	–	↔
Dihydro-2H-pyran-2-one (5,6-)	–	↔

Data are taken from Garle and Fry (1988), Fry *et al.* (1992), Wilkinson and Fry (1996), and M.J. Garle (unpublished observations). The reader is referred to these first three references for further details.

which no data are available) have been demonstrated to cause toxicity *in vivo* or *in vitro*, albeit in some cases under extreme conditions (i.e. prior depletion of cellular GSH).

2. The known species differences in extent of covalent binding of the paracetamol reactive metabolite to protein could be mimicked in this assay (Garle *et al.*, 1988).

3. For the compounds for which information is available, covalent binding to protein occurs via protein thiol groups. Iproniazid, which covalently binds to protein via a lysine residue, did not produce a positive response in this assay (Garle and Fry, 1988).

4. Substrates of the P450 system not believed to be metabolized to reactive metabolites (hexobarbitone, benzphetamine, aminopyrine, and biphenyl) produced a negative response (Garle and Fry, 1988).

5. Although run using liver microsomes, the assay was able to detect xenobiotics (4-ipomeanol, 3-methylindole, butylated hydroxytoluene) which typically produce extrahepatic metabolism-mediated toxicity *in vivo*, although a secondary liver toxicity has been observed under some circumstances with each of these xenobiotics.

6. Direct-acting GSH depletors could be readily discriminated from those that require metabolism, and the involvement of P450 in such metabolism-mediated GSH depletion could also be readily detected.

7. This assay has been used with human liver microsomes (Fry *et al.*, 1992). In principle, the assay could be used with any source of P450 (e.g. homogenates of cells stably transfected with individual P450 isoforms).

Taken together, these data suggest that such an assay could be useful for the detection of xenobiotics that exert their toxicity through reactive metabolites, but by itself gives no indication of the likely target-organ (although it would be one which has P450 activity) or even that toxicity will occur by this mechanism *in vivo*. The finding of a positive response in this assay would flag up a hazard warning; other information, possibly based on *in vitro* models of selective cytotoxicity, would be required to assess the risk from this hazard. It may be, given the size of the chemical library being screened, that a hazard warning flag is all that is required at this stage of screening. It should be a relatively straightforward matter to adapt such an approach for a HTS application. Other authors have utilized this idea of GSH trapping as the basis of an assay for reactive metabolites (Mulder and Le, 1988; Palmen and Evelo, 1993).

Xenobiotics may also exert toxicity through an oxidative stress mechanism (Scheme B in Figure 3.1), which also is associated with loss of GSH, in this case through its oxidation to the dimer glutathione disulphide (GSSG). In this mechanism, the xenobiotic undergoes a 1-electron reduction to yield a radical. This radical species can then be oxidized back to the parent compound ('redox cycling') at the expense of molecular oxygen, which is converted to superoxide anion radical and thence hydrogen peroxide. The hydrogen peroxide can be converted to water, at which stage GSH is oxidized to GSSG under the influence of glutathione peroxidase. At high rates of superoxide generation, the

> An assay could be useful for the detection of xenobiotics that exert their toxicity through reactive metabolites, but by itself gives no indication of the likely target organ or even that toxicity will occur by this mechanism *in vivo*.

regeneration of GSH from GSSG, by the action of glutathione reductase, cannot be maintained and oxidative stress ensues from the deleterious effects of the reactive oxygen species, in particular the hydroxyl radical (OH·).

Reductases capable of carrying out the initial 1-electron reduction of suitable xenobiotics also exist in the microsomal fraction so that the GSH depletion assay system has the potential to detect xenobiotics that exert toxicity through an oxidative stress mechanism, as exemplified by the positive response obtained with menadione, an archetypal redox cycler (Table 3.1).

Approaches such as that outlined above should prove attractive options for development of HTS for toxicity, in that they have a clear mechanistic basis, with good historical information (required for method validation), and are amenable to miniaturization and automation. However, it is worth re-emphasizing that this type of approach will only detect one, or at most two, mechanisms of toxicity, so that the aim should be to target for the most common modes of toxicity and accepting that rarer mechanisms will not be detected at this stage.

A further advantage to this type of approach is that its rationale is well accepted by toxicologists as it bears may similarities to the Ames test for bacterial mutagens: a) it has a well-defined mechanistic basis; b) it identifies potential toxic xenobiotics, but in itself gives no indication of likely target-organ; and c) it uses a metabolizing system comparable to that used in the Ames test.

3.5 Conclusions

The emphasis of this chapter has been on the use of existing technologies in aiding the establishment of toxicity profiles of new chemical entities in the context of HTS. From the foregoing discussion it should be apparent that no single test will satisfactorily define this toxicity profile, and that some aspects of cytotoxicity are currently not amenable to study in a high throughput mode. This leads on to the question of how to integrate the existing approaches, and to pose some suggestions for future work which would further the goal of devising meaningful HTS toxicity screens.

For the present, measurement of basal cytotoxicity, coupled with mechanistically-based tests along the lines described, appears to offer the best current approach. These assays are amenable to HTS and could be run in parallel, with the option of performing *in vitro* target-organ assays on the

QSAR for non-genotoxic systemic toxicity could be used at a very early stage of drug development. Various 'structural alerts' for such toxicity could act as starting points for this research.

reduced number of samples that emerge from this initial toxicity screen, to provide more detailed information.

For the future, it is to be hoped that efforts will be concentrated on developing QSAR for non-genotoxic systemic toxicity which could be used at a very early stage of drug development. Various 'structural alerts' for such toxicity are already apparent (e.g. quinones, epoxides, quinone-imines, etc.) which could act as starting points for this research. In addition, further fundamental research into the mechanisms underlying toxicity are essential to provide the theoretical framework on which develop new mechanistically-based tests; it is likely that this research will focus, in particular, on genomic alterations and cellular defence responses, which are the topic of some of the following chapters.

Acknowledgements

The author wishes to thank colleagues within FRAME (Fund for Replacement of Animals in Medical Experiments) and the pharmaceutical industry for the many stimulating discussions which have helped formulate the ideas presented in this chapter, and the industrial sponsors of FRAME for providing financial support for his own work.

References

Aikawa, K., Satoh, T., Kobayashi, K. and Kitagawa, H., 1978, Glutathione depletion by aniline analogs in vitro associated with liver microsomal cytochrome P450. *Japanese Journal of Pharmacology*, **28**, 699–705.

Atterwill, C.K. *et al.*, 1994, *In vitro* neurotoxicity testing, *ATLA*, **22**, 350–362.

Barile, F.A., Dierickx, P.J. and Kristen, U., 1994, In vitro cytotoxicity testing for prediction of acute human toxicity, *Cell Biology and Toxicology*, **10**, 155–162.

Blaauboer, B.J. *et al.*, 1994, The practical applicability of hepatocyte cultures in routine testing, *ATLA*, **22**, 231–241.

Brown, N.A. *et al.*, 1995, Screening chemicals for reproductive toxicity: the current alternatives, *ATLA*, **23**, 868–882.

Clemedson, C. *et al.*, 1996, MEIC evaluation of acute systemic toxicity. Part II. In vitro results from 68 toxicity assays used to test the first 30 reference chemicals and a comparative cytotoxicity analysis, *ATLA*, **24**, 273–311.

Cohen, S.D., Pumford, N.R., Khairallah, E.A., Boekelheide, K., Pohl, L.R., Amouzadeh, H.R. *et al.*, 1997, Selective protein covalent binding and target organ toxicity, *Toxicology and Applied Pharmacology*, **143**, 1–12.

Fry, J.R., 1992, Development in in vitro toxicology, *Comparative Haematology International*, **3**, 4–7.

Fry, J.R., Garle, M.J. and Hammond, A.H., 1988, Choice of acute toxicity measures for comparison of *in vivo/in vitro* toxicity, *ATLA*, **16**, 175–179.

Fry, J.R., Garle, M.J., Hammond, A.H. and Hatfield, A., 1990, Correlation of acute lethal potency with *in vitro* cytotoxicity, *Toxicology in Vitro*, **4**, 175–178.

Fry, J.R., Fentem, J.H., Salim, A., Tang, S.P.A., Garle, M.J. and Whiting, D.R., 1993, Structural requirements for the direct and cytochrome P450-dependent reaction of cyclic α,β- unsaturated carbonyl compounds with glutathione: a study with coumarin and related compounds, *Journal of Pharmacy and Pharmacology*, **45**, 166–170.

Garle, M.J. and Fry, J.R., 1988, Detection of reactive metabolites in vitro, *Toxicology*, **54**, 101–110.

Garle, M.J. and Fry, J.R., 1996, A comparison of hepatic enzyme activities and their modulation by dexamethazone in freshly isolated and cultured hepatocytes and in the differentiated hepatoma cell line, 2sFou, *ATLA*, **24**, 31–37.

Garle, M.J., Fentem, J.H. and Fry, J.R., 1994, *In vitro* cytotoxicity tests for the prediction of acute toxicity *in vivo*, *Toxicology in Vitro*, **8**, 1303–1312.

Garle, M.J., Khan, J. and Fry, J.R., 1988, Depletion of glutathione by the hepatotoxins paracetamol and bromobenzene, and their non-hepatotoxic analogues, in a fortified liver microsomal system, *Toxicology in Vitro*, **2**, 247–252.

Gribaldo, L. *et al.*, 1996, The use of *in vitro* systems for evaluating haematotoxicity, *ATLA*, **24**, 211–231.

Guzzie, P.J., 1994, Lethality testing, in Gad, S.C. (ed.), *In Vitro Toxicology*, New York: Raven Press, pp. 57–86.

Järkelid, L., Kjellstrand, P., Martinson, E. and Wieslander, A., 1997, Toxicity of 20 chemicals from the MEIC programme determined by growth inhibition of L-929 fibroblast-like cells, *ATLA*, **25**, 55–59.

Morin, J.-P., De Broe, M.E., Pfaller, W. and Schmuck, G., 1997, Nephrotoxicity testing *in vitro*: the current situation, *ATLA*, **25**, 497–503.

Mulder, G.J. and Le, C.T., 1988, A rapid, simple *in vitro* screening test, using [^{3}H]glutathione and L-[^{35}S]cysteine as trapping agents, to detect reactive intermediates of xenobiotics, *Toxicology in Vitro*, **2**, 225–230.

Nelson, S.D. and Pearson, P.G., 1990, Covalent and non-covalent interactions in acute lethal cell injury caused by chemicals, *Annual Review of Pharmacology and Toxicology*, **30**, 169–195.

Palmen, N.G.M. and Evelo, C.T.A., 1993, Glutathione depletion in human erythrocytes as an indicator for microsomal activation of cyclophosphamide and 3-hydroxyacetanilide, *Toxicology*, **84**, 157–170.

Seibert, H. *et al.*, 1996, Acute toxicity testing *in vitro* and the classification and labelling of chemicals, *ATLA*, **24**, 499–510.

Weiss, M.T. and Sawyer, T.W., 1993, Cytotoxicity of the MEIC test chemicals in primary neuron cultures, *Toxicology in Vitro*, **7**, 653–667.

Wilkinson, D.J. and Fry, J.R., 1995, Rat liver cytochrome P450-mediated metabolic activation of methoxsalen and structurally related compounds and its relation to enzyme inhibition, *Journal of Pharmacy and Pharmacology*, **47**, 79–84.

4 Gene Expression and its Applications to High Throughput Screens and Molecular Toxicology

Robert B. Burris, Robert T. Dunn II and Spencer B. Farr, Phase-1 Molecular Toxicology, Inc., Santa Fe, USA

4.1 Introduction

With the focus of the pharmaceutical industry directed toward moving larger numbers of clinically successful drugs through the development pipeline, the value of predicting toxicity by measuring gene expression patterns is being realized. The issues toxicologists are currently addressing are where the measurement of gene expression will be most useful and what is the best way to develop high throughput gene expression screening assays. Our understanding of changes in gene expression patterns is growing exponentially, driven largely by the advent of gene microarrays. This chapter includes an overview of parameters for the toxicologist to consider when developing high throughput gene expression assays, a description of relevant technologies, and an example of using rules to rank compounds for toxicity. A major goal of toxicogenomics is the identification of genes causally linked to specific toxicological outcomes, and we will focus on how different groups are discovering toxicologically relevant genes and how those genes are incorporated into high throughput toxicity screens (HTS).

A major goal of toxicogenomics is the identification of genes causally linked to specific toxicological outcomes, and how those genes are incorporated into high throughput toxicity screens (HTS).

4.2 The need for high throughput toxicity screens

There is an increasing number of potential drug candidates emerging from efficacy screens, due in large part to the screening of combinatorial chemical libraries. While the

"

concern that toxicology will be the bottleneck in drug development has not been fully realized, there remains a need for higher throughput assays to assess compound toxicity. The scientific goals of high throughput toxicity screens are not, at least initially, to significantly reduce the number of animal studies, but rather to ensure that the best compounds are advanced through to the *in vivo* phases of drug development. The cost of *in vivo* studies coupled with an increasing number of drug candidates and pressure to bring a larger number of new drugs to market has created the impetus for higher throughput screening assays. High throughput toxicity screens offer the advantages of significant savings in time and money and the potential to help prioritize lead compounds earlier in the drug development process. Prior to *in vivo* studies, screens are being employed to rank compounds for their probable toxic effects in animals. As structure–toxicity rules are developed and coupled with *in vitro* assays, compounds that have failed for toxicity reasons may be modified to retain efficacy and reduce toxicity.

As structure–toxicity rules are developed and coupled with *in vitro* assays, compounds that have failed for toxicity reasons may be modified to retain efficacy and reduce toxicity.

4.3 The advent of gene microarrays and their impact on toxicology

Recent technological advances in the field of high-density gene microarrays are having a dramatic impact on molecular toxicology. As is often the case with technologies today, glass-slide based microarrays themselves may have a short 'half-life' and a number of alternatives are already being developed. Some of these alternatives boast higher throughputs than microarrays and lower experimental costs. Regardless, no other technology has had the impact on drug discovery and toxicology that gene microarrays have. Therefore, this discussion of high-density gene expression measurement will be limited to microarrays, with the understanding that, within the context of measuring patterns of gene expression, any robust, multiplex method of measuring gene expression will also be valid. If one assumes the tenet that no toxicological event (with the possible exception of rapid necrosis) can occur without changes in gene expression patterns, the use of gene arrays in molecular toxicology will be pervasive for the foreseeable future. As recently as five years ago, the standard approach for measuring gene expression was Northern blot technology. The number of genes that could be measured in a single experiment was limited to several genes (assuming multiple

If one assumes the tenet that no toxicological event (with the possible exception of rapid necrosis) can occur without changes in gene expression patterns, the use of gene arrays in molecular toxicology will be pervasive for the foreseeable future.

Figure 4.1
Pattern Analysis. Connecting gene expression with traditional toxicological outcomes.

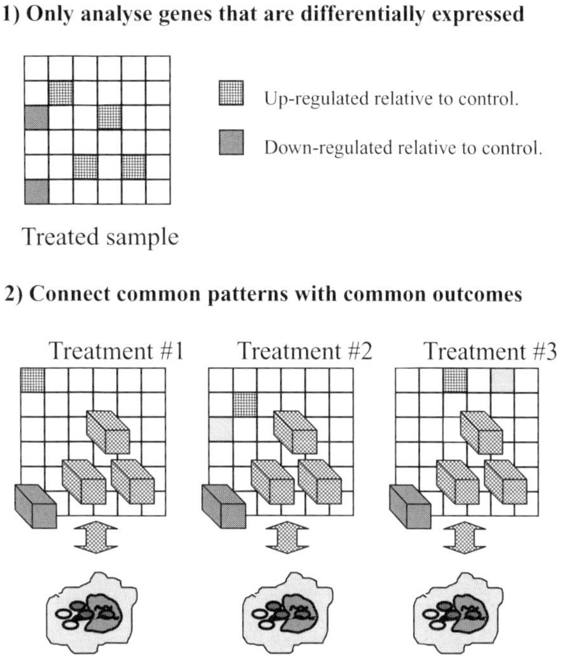

1) Only analyse genes that are differentially expressed

Up-regulated relative to control.

Down-regulated relative to control.

Treated sample

2) Connect common patterns with common outcomes

Treatment #1   Treatment #2   Treatment #3

strippings of the membrane). Now, the expression of tens of thousands of genes can be measured simultaneously on a single gene array. Studies that would previously have required years of labour to complete using Northern technology are now finished within a week. While discussions of gene arrays will be limited to their direct application to high throughput toxicity screening, they are likely to remain useful indefinitely for more in-depth analyses of *in vivo* studies. However, until the price of gene arrays drops dramatically, they will be cost-prohibitive for most groups in the screening of a large number of drug candidates. The development of high throughput toxicity screens is strengthened by the measurement of gene expression from *in vivo* studies; these are the studies where the connections between genes and toxic outcomes will be made (Figure 4.1). A better understanding of gene expression *in vivo* will facilitate the development of *in vitro* models for predicting human toxicity, a process already well underway.

The development of high throughput toxicity screens is strengthened by the measurement of gene expression from *in vivo* studies; these are the studies where the connections between genes and toxic outcomes will be made (Figure 4.1).

4.4 Developing high throughput gene expression toxicity screens

When developing predictive toxicity screens for ranking compounds, the toxicologist faces certain inherent challenges. These challenges are amplified when developing gene expression assays for high throughput toxicity screens, namely the investigator must initially design and run experiments to determine which genes are relevant to the endpoints of interest. In order to move gene expression into high throughput toxicity screening assays effectively, a number of issues must be addressed:

- Determine toxicologically relevant genes
- Place relevant genes on a microarray (or analogous system)
- Treat animals or cells with learning sets of compounds
- Derive rules based upon gene expression patterns
- Move relevant subset of genes into an higher throughput testing environment
- Validate gene expression for the appropriate *in vitro* model system (cell line, primary cell, etc.)

4.5 Finding toxicologically relevant genes

The amount of time and money spent determining which genes are relevant for toxicological endpoints of interest will likely exceed all other areas of development of high throughput screens combined. While the human genome is comprised of approximately 100,000 genes, it is estimated that only about 15,000 genes are expressed in any given cell, at any given time (Zhang *et al.*, 1997). Expression of many genes is limited to different stages of development and differentiation while other genes respond specifically to different types of toxic insults. When trying to connect gene expression with an organ specific toxic outcome, the challenge is to determine which of the 15,000 genes are toxicologically relevant.

There are two principal approaches for measuring toxicologically relevant gene expression. The first approach measures expression of a large number of genes by utilizing ESTs (Expressed-Sequence Tags, i.e. gene fragments generated from cDNA libraries), often measuring tens of thousands of genes per experiment. However, current estimates are that less than 50% of all human cDNA sequences are present in the public EST database (Welford *et al.*, 1998). Elucidating connections between gene expression and toxic effects is the cornerstone of the second approach. Experiments are

Three accepted methods for determining which genes are differentially expressed are differential display, SAGE (serial analysis of gene expression), and AFLP (amplified fixed-length polymorphisms).

designed with learning sets of compounds (compounds that elicit a diverse set of toxic outcomes) and differentially expressed genes are identified for each treatment. Previously uncharacterized genes can be sequenced, amplified, and spotted as targets on microarrays. Only after this process has been completed can new experiments be designed (i.e. testing a number of compounds that cause a common toxic outcome) to elucidate which genes are differentially expressed. Three accepted methods for determining which genes are differentially expressed are differential display, SAGE (serial analysis of gene expression), and AFLP (amplified fixed-length polymorphisms).

4.6 Differential display

Differential display (Liang *et al.*, 1992) has been used for the identification of genes that are differentially expressed in either different cell types or in a common cell type but under different toxic challenges.

Differential display (Liang *et al.*, 1992) has been used for the identification of genes that are differentially expressed in either different cell types or in a common cell type but under different toxic challenges (Fischer *et al.*, 1998; Donat and Abel, 1998; Damiani *et al.*, 1998; Walden *et al.*, 1998; Kocher *et al.*, 1995; Chen *et al.*, 1998a; Vanden Heuvel *et al.*, 1998; Schwahn *et al.*, 1998; Chen *et al.*, 1998b; Chan *et al.*, 1998; Harris *et al.*, 1998; Gupta *et al.*, 1998). Differential display utilizes the polymerase chain reaction (PCR) to separate and clone individual mRNAs (Figure 4.2). The success

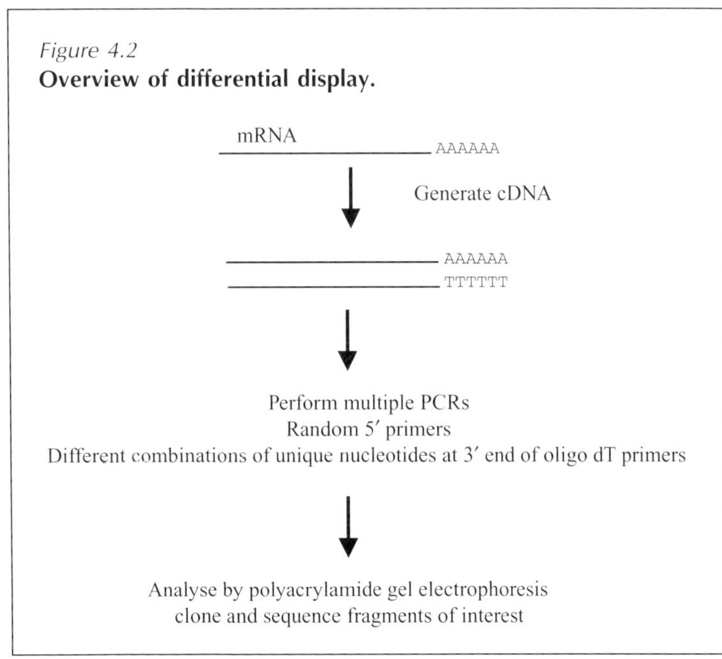

Figure 4.2
Overview of differential display.

of this methodology rests in the choice of oligonucleotide primers to generate unique cDNA fragments. The 3′ PCR primers are anchored to the polyadenylated tail by a short stretch of thymidine residues, followed by unique combinations of nucleotides at the 3′ end. There are 12 possible combinations of the last two 3′ bases with the caveat that thymidine cannot be the second to last base. The 5′ PCR primers are short and their sequences arbitrary. Two different mRNA populations (treated and untreated) are amplified independently using the same set of primers and compared on sequencing gels. Differentially expressed genes are identified, cloned, and sequenced. Differential display is considered to be more qualitative in nature (Ledakis *et al.*, 1998) than either SAGE or AFLP (i.e. differential display can determine which genes are differentially expressed but not to what extent).

4.7   SAGE

Serial analysis of gene expression (SAGE) is capable of identifying novel genes and quantifying relative abundance of differentially expressed transcripts (Velculescu *et al.*, 1995; Madden *et al.*, 1997; Hibi *et al.*, 1998). This methodology generates short characteristic 'tags' that are concatenated, cloned, and sequenced, thereby generating expression information for multiple genes simultaneously (Figure 4.3). In the initial step, an mRNA population is reverse transcribed with a biotinylated oligo-dT primer. Cleavage of the resulting cDNA by an anchoring enzyme generates a pool of DNA fragments. An anchoring enzyme is a restriction enzyme, usually with a four base pair recognition site; a four base pair recognition site is sufficient to cut most transcripts at least once. Biotinylated groups on the oligo-dT primer allow isolation of 3′ cDNA fragments by binding to streptavidin beads. The cDNA/streptavidin complex is then divided in half and each half is ligated to a different linker (A and B). A tagging enzyme (a restriction enzyme that generates blunt-end fragments a fixed distance from the recognition site) cleaves the cDNA fragments. Resulting 'primer A' fragments and 'primer B' fragments are blunt end ligated to each other and amplified with primers A and B, generating 'ditags' (two small sequence fragments, one each from a 'primer A' fragment and a 'primer B' fragment). Cleavage of this ligation product by the anchoring enzyme results in ditags flanked on each end by the anchoring enzyme restriction sites. Ditags are concatenated, cloned, and eventually sequenced. Sequencing concatemers is the most labour intensive part of the process.

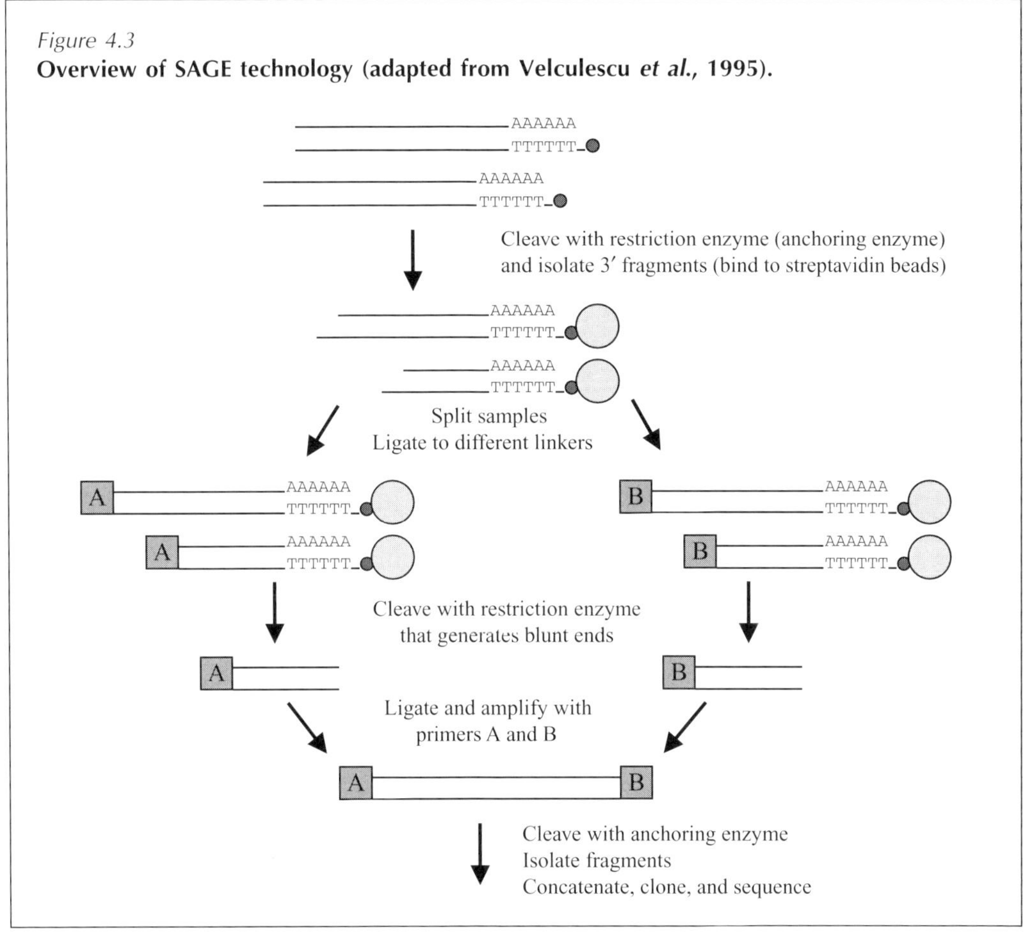

Figure 4.3
Overview of SAGE technology (adapted from Velculescu *et al.*, 1995).

4.8 AFLP

AFLP (amplified fragment length polymorphism) methodology is available from Perkin Elmer Genscope and utilizes both restriction digestion and PCR.

AFLP (amplified fragment length polymorphism) methodology is available from Perkin Elmer Genscope and utilizes both restriction digestion and PCR (Figure 4.4) (Hong *et al.*, 1998; Habu *et al.*, 1997; Money *et al.*, 1996). Initially, mRNA is reverse transcribed into double stranded cDNA. cDNA fragments are digested with *Eco*RI (or another restriction enzyme with a six base-pair recognition site) and fragments most proximal to the 3′ end of the gene are isolated from the remaining fragments. *Mse*I (or another restriction enzyme with a four base-pair recognition site) cleaves these 3′ fragments and oligonucleotide adapters, containing *Eco*RI and *Mse*I sites, are ligated to the ends of these fragments. The oligonucleotide adapters are complementary to the PCR primers and the fluorescent label is incorporated into the *Eco*RI PCR primer so that only those fragments with *Eco*RI

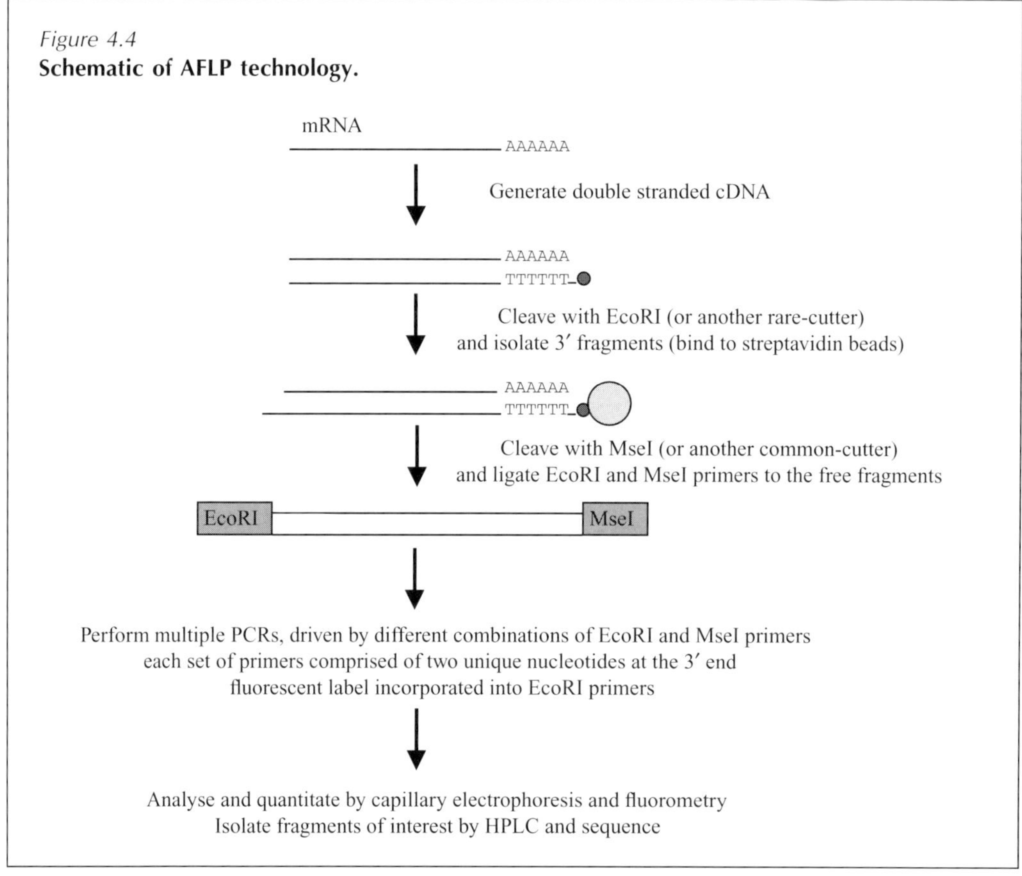

Figure 4.4
Schematic of AFLP technology.

and *Mse*I sites at either end are labelled by PCR. The small number of fragments that have *Mse*I sites at both ends are not fluorescently labelled during amplification. Reducing a large number of fragments down to more manageable numbers is accomplished by the number of unique nucleotides at the ends of the PCR primers. For example, four PCR primers for the *Eco*RI fragment can be selected each having a single unique nucleotide at the 3' end of the primer (G, A, T, or C). If the PCR primers for the *Mse*I end also have four unique nucleotides at their end, the number of gene fragments in any given pool has been reduced by a factor of approximately 16 (4 × 4). If there are 15,000 gene fragments, any given pool will contain approximately 15,000/16 or 937 fragments, a number too large to distinguish by capillary electrophoresis. However, if a PCR primer set containing all possible combinations of two unique nucleotides at the 3' end of both PCR primers is used, the number of fragments in any given reaction will be 15,000/256 or approximately 60, a number that can be distinguished readily by capillary electrophoresis. The greater the number of unique PCR primers, the greater the number of electrophoretic separations that must be performed. Most of the labour required to perform AFLP involves running individual capillary electrophoresis separations. As the use of 96-well capillary electrophoresis instrumentation becomes available, the amount of time required to analyse samples will be reduced significantly. One of the major advantages of this technology is that the scientist need analyse only genes that are differentially expressed. Gene fragments of interest are isolated by HPLC and then sequenced. Once a gene has been identified and analysed, it can be identified in subsequent analyses of new samples, thereby eliminating redundant analyses. This system is both quantitative and efficient.

4.9 Measuring toxicologically relevant genes with microarrays

Regardless of how toxicologically relevant genes are identified, the next step in the process is to engineer a microarray that contains the genes of interest. DNA targets attached to the slide can either be synthesized on the surface of the slide (Affymetrix' photolithography methodology) or, more commonly, the DNA is chemically attached to the slide (Figure 4.5). DNA used in this chemical attachment is usually the PCR product of a cloned gene, although various groups continue to work on the development of attachment chemistries for the specific attachment at a 5' or 3' modified terminus.

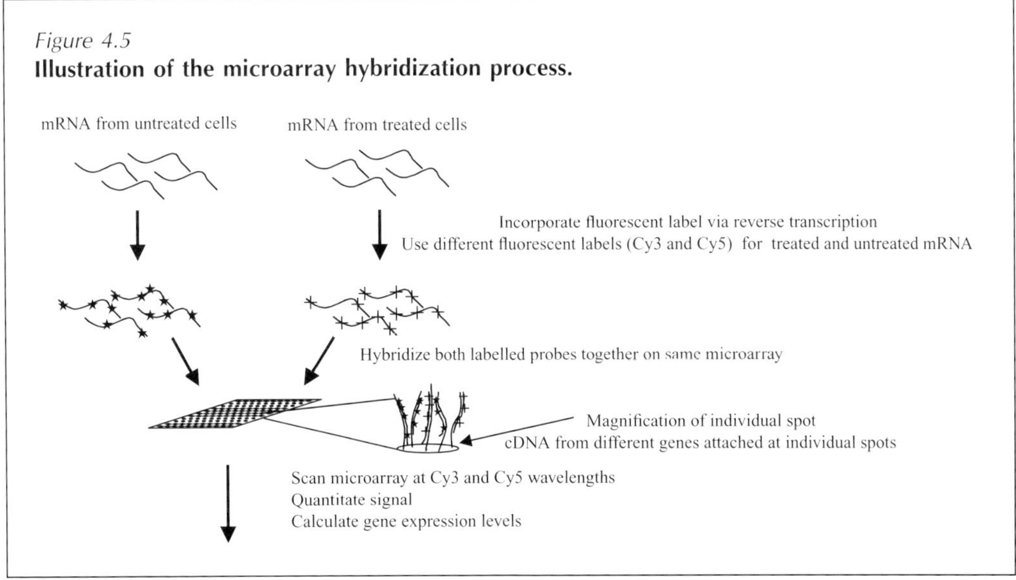

Figure 4.5
Illustration of the microarray hybridization process.

Figure 4.6
Sensitivity vs specificity. A given gene may be highly sensitive to agents that share a common toxicologically relevant outcome. However, if that gene is also induced by a significant number of agents that do not share that outcome, then induction of that gene will not be a good predictor of that outcome.

Compound	DNA Damage	c-FOS
MMS	yes	up
MNNG	yes	up
EMS	yes	up
Mitomycin C	yes	up
Actinomycin D	yes	up
UVC	yes	up
Serum	no	up
EGF	no	up
PDGF	no	up
NGF	no	up
IL-2	no	up
IL-6	no	up
cAMP	no	up
TPA	no	up

4.10 Devising strategies for deriving toxicity rules

The choice of a learning set of compounds is important for deriving a valid set of rules for predicting a desired endpoint. Clearly, a sufficiently large set of 'positive' compounds (compounds that elicit the desired toxic effect) is required to be able to find the genes that correlate with the toxicologically relevant outcome. The choice of 'negative' compounds (compounds that do not elicit the desired toxic effect) is also critically important. Compounds that do not cause the toxic response of interest are necessary to eliminate genes that are not specific for the toxicity outcome, i.e. genes that respond to both the 'positive' compounds and 'negative' compounds (Figure 4.6). When selecting a learning set of compounds, care should be given to ensure that the compounds are relevant to the field of interest. Different sets of compounds are likely to be used to derive rules for the environmental sector versus the pharmaceutical industry. The 'negative' set of compounds should be representative and sufficiently large for the field of interest. Additionally, a number of groups are testing structurally diverse sets of compounds,

The choice of a learning set of compounds is important for deriving a valid set of rules for predicting a desired endpoint. After the learning set of compounds has been chosen, either animals or cells are dosed, gene expression is measured, and the data entered into a bioinformatics system capable of deriving ranking rules.

with the belief that the resultant data can eventually empower structure–toxicity relationship rules.

After the learning set of compounds has been chosen, either animals or cells are dosed, gene expression is measured, and the data entered into a bioinformatics system capable of deriving ranking rules. The process of challenging cells or animals with compounds, measuring gene expression, and analysing data to determine rules is likely to be an iterative process. Gene expression should initially be measured in concert with other toxicologically relevant endpoints (e.g. blood serum chemistry, histopathology), whether at the cellular level, the organ level, or the whole animal level. Comparisons are made between compounds at doses that elicit similar responses in other relevant toxicological endpoints. When doses are chosen that have either no effect or are extremely toxic, the amount of useful information is diminished.

Connecting gene expression patterns from a cell culture system with traditional *in vivo* and human endpoints is more associative in nature. The gene expression patterns are not connected directly with the outcome in question, but rather associations are made between patterns of gene expression and toxic outcomes. When comparing compounds, care should be taken to ensure that gene expression is measured at comparable levels of cellular 'stress' (e.g. within a defined range of cytotoxicity) to ensure that valid comparisons are made.

4.11 Deriving gene expression/toxicity rules

Unless the number of compounds tested is extremely large, it is probable that a large number of putative predictive rules will be derived from gene microarray studies. Many of these rules will be invalid and the investigator is left to rely upon judgement to determine which rule sets are actually valid. It is probable that the different groups involved in this process will need to couple expert judgement with statistical analyses to develop rules connected with the relevant outcome. Thus, the need for input from toxicologists with an understanding of the relationship between gene expression and cellular outcomes remains. A number of groups are using statistical analysis packages to evaluate data. Software packages from companies like StatSoft, SAS, etc. are being used because, within a single software package, a number of different analyses can be examined. Analyses like principal components, classification trees, and discriminant analysis are being used to glean toxicologically relevant genes from complex data sets.

4.12 High throughput gene expression systems

A number of higher throughput systems are available for analysing gene expression from native mRNA transcripts. These systems are not based upon reporter construct technologies and, therefore, are applicable to a wider range of cell types and animal tissues. Among these systems are the CytoStar-T™ *in situ* mRNA assay (Amersham/Pharmacia), TaqMan™ (Perkin Elmer), and branched DNA (Chiron). Each assay has its own unique advantages and limitations. All of these gene expression assays are most feasible, with respect to throughput, when a limited number of genes (<20) are measured.

4.12.1 *CytoStar-T*™ in situ *gene expression assay*

The CytoStar-T™ *in situ* gene expression assay (Harris *et al.*, 1996) is based upon technology in which scintillants are embedded into the polystyrene base of 96-well tissue culture microplates (Figure 4.7) (Graves *et al.*, 1997). When radioisotopes with suitable decay characteristics are brought into close proximity with the scintillant-containing base, light is generated and measured by a 96-well plate scintillation

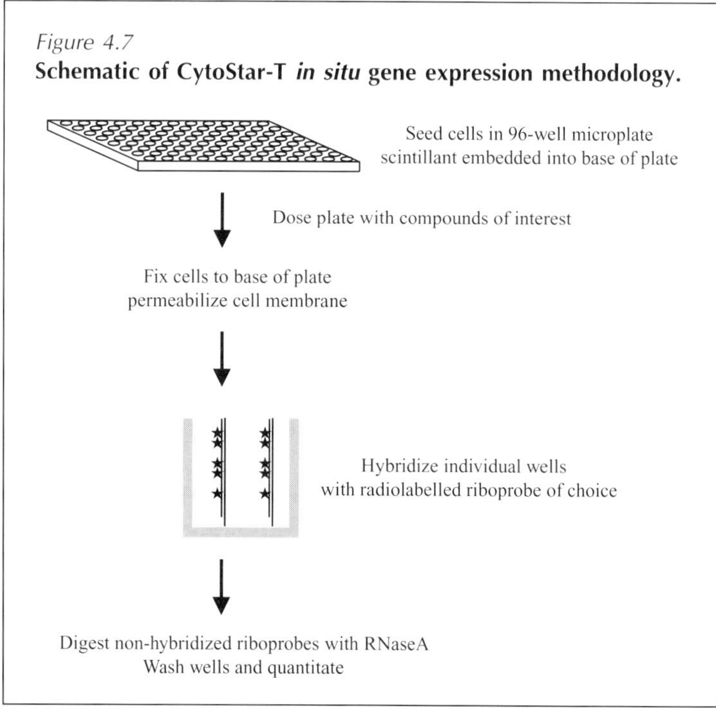

Figure 4.7
Schematic of CytoStar-T *in situ* gene expression methodology.

counter. It is required that cells adhere to the base of the microplate in this assay and either cell lines or primary cells can be used. Cells are challenged with the compound of interest and, after the desired exposure, cells are permeabilized and formalin fixed to the base of the plate. [^{33}P]-labelled riboprobes are generated from an *in vitro* transcription reaction with each riboprobe complementary and specific to a gene of interest. The riboprobe for the gene of interest is introduced into the well and allowed to hybridize to its complementary mRNA. Ribonuclease A is added to the wells, non-hybridized probes are degraded, the wells are washed, and the amount of hybridized riboprobe is measured in a 96-well plate scintillation counter. In this manner, the expression of a number of genes can be monitored simultaneously. Data generated in this assay have low coefficients of variation and results are highly reproducible.

4.12.2 *Branched DNA (bDNA)*

In contrast to PCR-based nucleic acid detection technologies that rely on enzymatic amplification of target sequences, Chiron Corporation's bDNA detection system relies on signal amplification of physiological levels of mRNA through a series of hybridizations of target sequence to various oligonucleotide probes (Figure 4.8). The details of the bDNA technology have been described in detail elsewhere (Urdea, 1994; Wang *et al.*, 1997). Essential features of the bDNA assay include hybridization of the target sequence to capture probes that are bound to 96-well assay microplates and hybridization of target to label probes complementary to both the target sequences and a part of the bDNA molecule. A second hybridization takes place that involves binding of bDNA molecules to regions of the label probes. Finally, an alkaline phosphatase-labelled oligonucleotide, complementary to regions of the bDNA molecule, is added to the well, followed by addition of an alkaline phosphatase substrate and luminescent detection. The bDNA assay requires synthesis of numerous oligonucleotide probes in order to permit signal amplification. In a study of the regulation of insulin mRNA splicing, ten separate oligonucleotide probes were used to detect murine insulin mRNA (Wang *et al.*, 1997). The bDNA assay does not rely on enzymatic amplification of a target sequence(s) and is not as sensitive as PCR-based techniques (Wang *et al.*, 1997). However, the bDNA assay is more quantitatively reproducible than PCR-based systems. The bDNA assay has found utility in the estimation of viral load in patients with hepatitis B and C as well as HIV

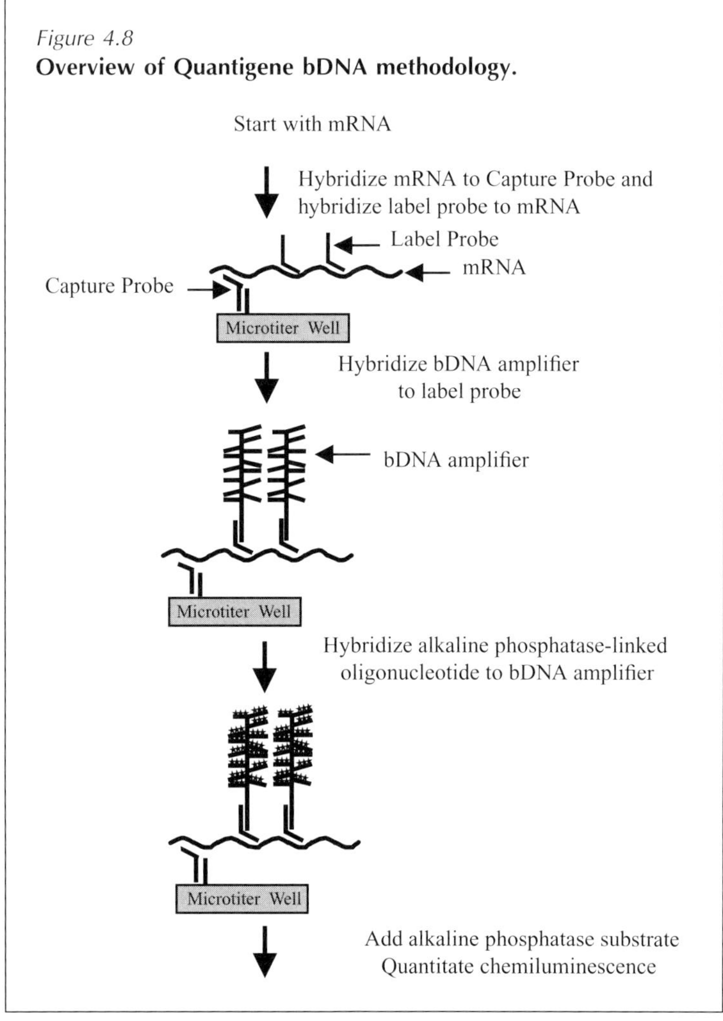

(Urdea, 1994; Todd *et al.*, 1995). The similarity of the bDNA assay format, called Quantigene™, to an ELISA-type system enables the bDNA assay to function as a moderately high throughput tool for monitoring gene expression.

4.12.3 *TaqMan*™

Nucleic acid quantitation during PCR is most valid during early cycles of PCR when none of the reagents have become limiting. The first quantitative PCR systems utilized intercalator dyes such as ethidium bromide to quantitate accumulation of PCR product (Higuchi *et al.*, 1992; 1993). The weakness of this approach was that the system could not distinguish between specific and nonspecific PCR products. A recent advancement has come from using specific oligonucleotide probes (20–30 nucleotides in length) that have attached reporter and quencher dyes within the same oligonucleotide molecule. These labelled probes are designed to hybridize to a part of the target sequence internal to the PCR primers. When these oligonucleotides are intact, the fluorescence of the reporter moiety is quenched due to fluorescent resonance energy transfer (FRET) between reporter and quencher (Heid *et al.*, 1996). The TaqMan™ PCR detection system utilizes the 5′ exonuclease activity of Taq polymerase. As the Taq polymerase catalyzes primer extension, its 5′ exonuclease activity cleaves the internal probe which releases the fluorescent dye. Once the fluorescent dye is free in solution, its fluorescence is no longer quenched and signal can be detected with the Applied Biosystem 7700 analytical PCR and sequence detector. The amount of reporter dye released is proportional to the amount of nucleic acid present in the reaction. The fluorescence data are compared to a standard curve that permits estimation of initial copy number of the target being measured. The TaqMan™ system utilizes a 96-well format and is thus amenable to high throughput analysis of differences in gene expression. The commercially available TaqMan™ system is able to measure template amplification directly within the reaction tube.

4.13   Reporter constructs

For certain types of toxic events, reporter systems may be appropriate for prioritizing compounds. A reporter construct is created by fusing the promoter (or a response element) from a gene of interest to the coding region of a reporter gene. For high throughput screening systems, reporter constructs are usually stably transfected into cell lines. Reporter constructs are most often co-transfected into cell lines with an antibiotic resistance gene, for purposes of selecting viable clones. Reporter systems, with all their inherent limitations (i.e. reduced metabolic functions, cell cycle deregulation, etc.), offer the highest throughput for the measurement of gene expression. The caveat with reporter systems is that the investigator must know the limitations of the cell line (or cell type) they are working with. Two reporter systems (green fluorescent protein and luciferase) are discussed below.

4.13.1   *Green fluorescent protein*

The isolation of green fluorescent protein (GFP) from the jellyfish *Aequorea victoria* was reported in 1962 (Shimomura *et al.*, 1962). Sensitivity has always been a disadvantage with GFP, but recent advances in GFP technology address these sensitivity issues. Mutant GFPs have been created that are brighter than wild-type GFP and microplate fluorometers have been developed that detect lower amounts of fluorescence. The need for the development of brighter mutants for a microplate GFP assay comes from the inherent lack of sensitivity of the wild-type gene. This is especially problematic for the toxicologist where many of the genes of interest are low expressor genes induced only under conditions of stress. Data often couldn't be generated for untreated cells, a prerequisite for determining fold induction. Advantages of the GFP system are that it is non-invasive, requires no substrate, and GFP is a stable protein that will accumulate for monitoring purposes. Additionally, GFP's chromophore is formed from an internal portion of the primary sequence of GFP (Phe64-Ser-Tyr-Gly-Val-Gln69) and, thus, does not dissociate. As issues in sensitivity are overcome, this system may become one of the highest throughput gene expression reporter systems.

4.13.2 *Luciferase*

Reporter constructs that utilize luciferase can be adapted for use as screening systems in toxicology. Luciferase technology relies on the activity of luciferase enzyme and its ability to oxidize luciferin. Luciferin oxidation leads to the emission of light energy that can be readily measured. Systems based upon luciferase have several key advantages:

- detection is non-radioactive
- increased sensitivity over CAT-based (chloramphenicol acetyl transferase) systems
- numerous vectors are available that enable testing promoter/enhancer regions for genes of interest (Promega)

Luciferase reporter systems have already become useful for toxicology. The effects of certain metals on promoter function have been utilized by linking the PEPCK promoter to a luciferase reporter construct (Hamilton *et al.*, 1998). Luciferase-based reporter systems have also been used to define promoter regions of the organic anion transporting polypeptide (OATP) (Kullak-Ublick *et al.*, 1997). Finally, responsiveness of cells and genes to 2,3,7,8-TCDD and other halogenated aromatic hydrocarbons have been defined, in part, by luciferase systems (Walsh *et al.*, 1996; Murk *et al.*, 1996; Hoffer *et al.*, 1996).

4.14 Validating gene expression/toxicity rules

There is a growing interest in developing cell lines that are metabolically competent, eliminating the need for a bioactivation step.

As the measurement of gene expression becomes increasingly more common and genes associated with toxic outcomes become better defined, the emphasis for developing high throughput assays will shift toward finding cell lines or cell types which more accurately reflect the endpoint of interest. There is a growing interest in developing cell lines that are metabolically competent, eliminating the need for a bioactivation step.

4.15 Ranking compounds for genotoxicity

An example of how the toxicologist can select genes connected with a given endpoint (in this case, genotoxicity), move those genes into a high throughput assay, devise a set of rules, test compounds, and rank compounds for genotoxicity will be described in this section. In this study, the system used to measure gene expression was the CytoStar-T™ *in situ* mRNA assay from Amersham. Genes measured in this study were not selected from a comprehensive gene microarray analysis, as discussed previously, but instead were selected from the literature. Genes measured in this study were c-fos, c-myc, gadd45, gadd153, c-jun, bax, c-abl, and waf-1. β-actin was also measured and served as the housekeeping gene for normalization of treated samples to controls. Fold induction was calculated as follows (gadd45 serves as an example):

$$\text{Fold induction (gadd45)} = \frac{\dfrac{\text{gadd45 cpm (treated cells)}}{\text{gadd45 cpm (control cells)}}}{\dfrac{\beta\text{-actin cpm (treated cells)}}{\beta\text{-actin cpm (control cells)}}}$$

where the units 'cpm' are counts per minute, the output reading from a 96-well scintillation counter. Rules for predicting genotoxicity are based upon a percentage of maximum fold induction and are derived as follows (again using gadd45 as the example gene):

- For gadd45, determine which compound resulted in its largest fold induction. This fold induction serves as the maximum fold induction for gadd45 (Figure 4.9). This process is repeated for each gene.
- For all compounds, divide the fold induction for gadd45 by the maximum fold induction for gadd45. Repeat this process for each gene. For each compound, every gene

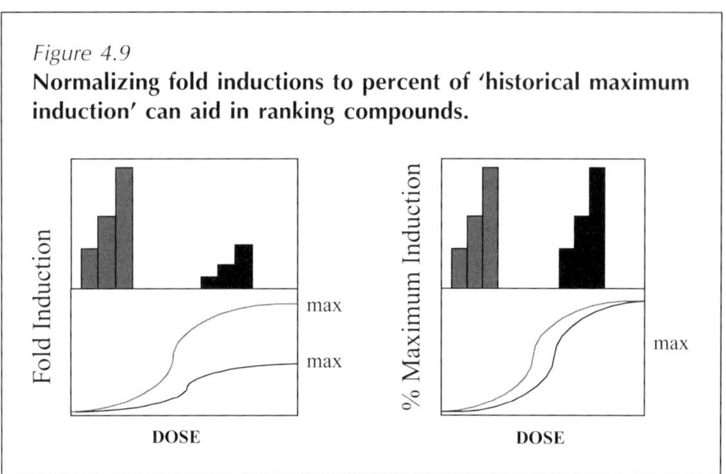

Figure 4.9
Normalizing fold inductions to percent of 'historical maximum induction' can aid in ranking compounds.

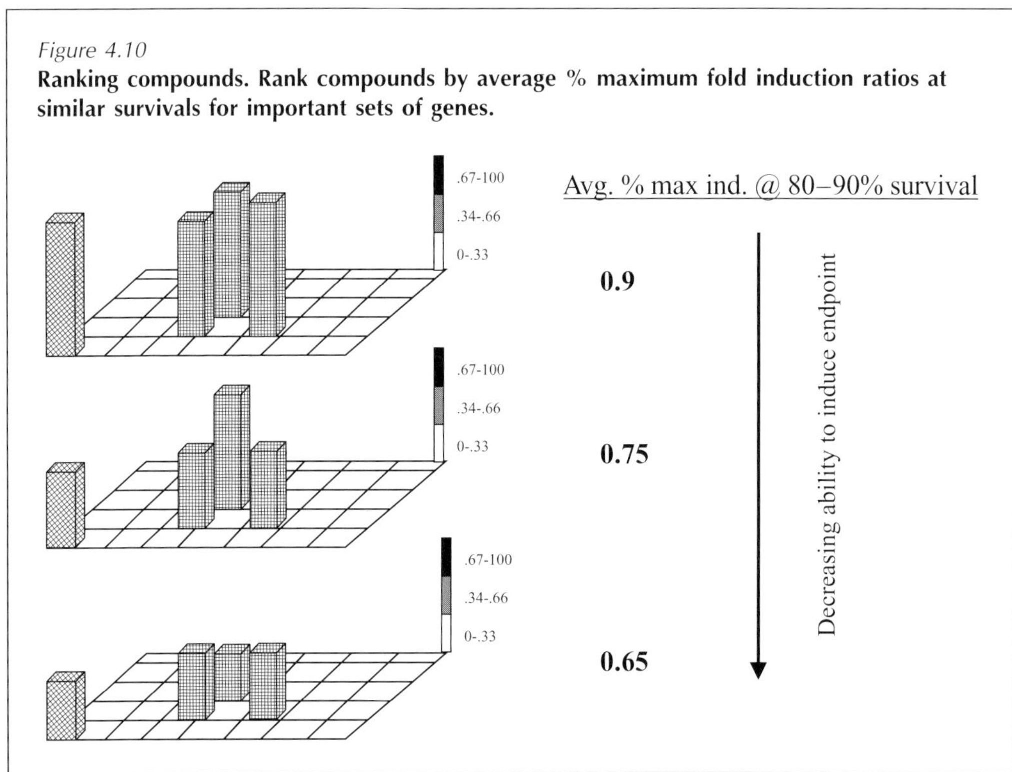

Figure 4.10
Ranking compounds. Rank compounds by average % maximum fold induction ratios at similar survivals for important sets of genes.

now has a value that is the percent of maximum fold induction.

- For each compound, calculate the average of the maximum fold inductions for all genes.
- Rank compounds. Compounds with the highest average maximum fold induction are considered the most genotoxic (Figure 4.10).

Figure 4.11

Ranking compounds. Ranking compounds by % maximum fold induction compares favourably with other traditional genotoxicity endpoints.

CHEMICAL	Concentration	AVG. % MAX IND.	Rodent Carc.	SCE	AMES	LD50 Mouse
PMA	25 µg/ml	**62.2%**	Pos	Pos	**Neg**	?
MMS	50 µg/ml	**52.9%**	Pos	Pos	Pos	290 mg/kg
Streptozotocin	1.2 mg/ml	**49.3%**	Pos	?	Pos	?
Mitomycin C	3.1 µg/ml	**38.5%**	Pos	Pos	Inconcl.	30 mg/kg
Carmustine	187.5 µg/ml	**31.7%**	Pos	?	?	19 mg/kg
Hydroxyurea	8.0 µg/ml	**12.9%**	**Neg**	**Neg**	?	7330 mg/kg
Acetominophen	40 µg/ml	**10.9%**	**Neg**	?	**Neg**	338 mg/kg

In this particular study, actinomycin D caused a 24 fold induction of gadd45, the largest induction observed for gadd45. Induction levels of gadd45 for all other compounds were normalized to this value. Dexamethasone was observed to cause a 1.25 fold induction of gadd45. The percent of maximum fold induction for dexamethasone was therefore 1.25/24 = 5.2%. These calculations were performed for all compounds and all genes and the averages of the % maximum fold induction for individual genes were calculated for all compounds. In our example, PMA had the highest average % maximum fold induction and, therefore, ranked as the most genotoxic compound (Figure 4.11). When performing the analyses, it became obvious that removing c-fos from the calculations did not affect the relative orders of compounds in the ranking scheme. Why was this? The answer lies in the issue of sensitivity vs. specificity. As was observed in Figure 4.6, c-fos not only responds to genotoxic compounds, but also responds to a wide-spectrum of non-genotoxic compounds. The result is that c-fos does not contribute to the predictive accuracy of the ranking scheme. The more genes included in the ranking scheme that are not specific for genotoxicity, the less accurate the ranking of compounds. In addition, the consideration of drug absorption, metabolism, and efficacy data can further refine the ranking of compounds.

4.16 Conclusions

There exists the very real possibility that larger numbers of efficacious new chemical entities will emerge from combinatorial chemical libraries within the pharmaceutical industry. The increase in potentially viable compounds while

Toxicologists are beginning to avail themselves to high throughput technologies and this process will minimize the potential for a bottleneck in the drug development process. Toxicologists must not lose sight of making connections between the results of high throughput screens for toxicity and classical organ and tissue specific toxicity endpoints such as cholestasis and nephrotoxicity.

beneficial in most respects (e.g. more potential good lead candidates) will pose a problem for toxicology. The demands in terms of resources and time to advance lead compounds through traditional preclinical toxicology may prevent advancement of truly good candidates that emerge from high throughput efficacy screens. Toxicologists are beginning to avail themselves to high throughput technologies and this process will minimize the potential for a bottleneck in the drug development process. In addition, toxicologists must not lose sight of making connections between the results of high throughput screens for toxicity and classical organ and tissue specific toxicity endpoints such as cholestasis and nephrotoxicity. The data coming out of gene expression studies are of very limited usefulness unless interpreted in the larger context of tissue, organ, and organismal toxicity. Now, for the first time, we can use the same technique to query gene expression at all levels of system complexity, resulting in the empowerment of high throughput, gene expression screens. In this way, high throughput gene expression screens, in the context of toxicology, may fulfil their mission of advancing the best lead candidates to more laborious and expensive preclinical studies.

References

Chan, E.C., Lue, M.Y., Hsu, K.C. and Fan, H.A., 1998, Identification of novel genes that are differentially expressed in human colorectal carcinoma, *Biochim. Biophys. Acta*, **1407**, 200–204.

Chen, C., Yin, X., Zhou, D., Shen, Z., Chi, C. and Gu, J., 1998a, Transcriptional regulation of human transcription factor IIB in SMMC-7721 human hepatocellular carcinoma cells by all-trans-retinoic acid and phorbol 12-myristate 13-acetate, *J. Cancer Res. Clin. Oncol.*, **124**, 493–496.

Chen, F.W., Davies, J.P. and Ioannou, Y.A., 1998b, Differential gene expression in apoptosis: identification of ribosomal protein 23K, a cell proliferation inhibitor, *Mol. Genet. Metab.*, **64**, 271–282.

Damiani, G., Capelli, E., Comincini, S., Mori, E., Panelli, S. and Cuccia, M., 1998, Identification of mRNAs differentially expressed in lymphocytes following interleukin-2 activation, *Exp. Cell Res.*, **245**, 27–33.

Donat, S. and Abel, J., 1998, Analysis of gene expression in lung and thymus of TCDD treated C57BL/6 mice using differential display RT-PCR, *Chemosphere*, **37**, 1867–1872.

Fischer, V., Schmitt, U., Weigmann, H., Keller, B., Reuss, S., Hiemke, C. *et al.*, 1998, Chronical haloperidol and clozapine treatment in rats: differential RNA display analysis, behavioral studies and serum level determination, *Prog. Neuropsychopharmacol. Biol. Psychiatry*, **22**, 1129–1139.

Graves, R., Davies, R., Brophy, G., O'Beirne, G. and Cook, N., 1997, Noninvasive, real-time method for the examination of thymidine uptake events – application of the method to V-79 cell synchrony studies, *Anal. Biochem.*, **248**, 251–257.

Gupta, R., Thomas, P., Beddington, R.S.P. and Rigby, P.W.J., 1998, Isolation of developmentally regulated genes by differential display screening of cDNA libraries, *Nucleic Acids Res.*, **26**, 4538–4539.

Habu, Y., Fukada-Tanaka, S., Hisatomi, Y. and Iida, S., 1997, Amplified restriction fragment length polymorphism-based mRNA fingerprinting using a single restriction enzyme that recognizes a 4-bp sequence, *Biochem. Biophys. Res. Commun.*, **234**, 516–521.

Hamilton, J.W., Kaltreider, R.C., Bajenova, O.V., Ihnat, M.A., McCaffrey, J., Turpie, B.W. *et al.*, 1998, Molecular basis for effects of carcinogenic heavy metals on inducible gene expression, *Environ Health Perspect.*, **106** Suppl 4, 1005–1015.

Harris, A.J., Shaddock, J.G., Manjanatha, M.G., Lisenbey, J.A. and Casciano, D.A., 1998, Identification of differentially expressed genes in aflatoxin B1-treated cultured primary rat hepatocytes and Fischer 344 rats, *Carcinogenesis*, **19**, 1451–1458.

Harris, D.W., Kenrick, M.K., Pither, R.J., Anson, J.G. and Jones, D.A., 1996, Development of a high-volume in situ mRNA hybridization assay for the quantification of gene expression utilizing scintillating microplates, *Anal. Biochem.*, **243**, 249–256.

Heid, C.A., Stevens, J., Livak, K.J. and Williams, P.M., 1996, Real time quantitative PCR, *Genome Res.*, **6**, 986–994.

Hibi, K., Liu, Q., Beaudry, G.A., Madden, S.L., Westra, W.H., Wehage, S.L. *et al.*, 1998, Serial analysis of gene expression in non-small cell lung cancer, *Cancer Res.*, **58**, 5690–5694.

Higuchi, R., Dollinger, G., Walsh, P.S. and Griffith, R., 1992, Simultaneous amplification and detection of specific DNA sequences, *Biotechnology*, **10**, 413–417.

Higuchi, R., Fockler, C., Dollinger, G. and Watson, R., 1993, Kinetic PCR analysis: real-time monitoring of DNA amplification reactions, *Biotechnology*, **11**, 1026–1030.

Hoffer, A., Chang, C.Y. and Puga, A., 1996, Dioxin induces transcription of fos and jun genes by Ah receptor-dependent and -independent pathways, *Toxicol. Appl. Pharmacol.*, **141**, 238–247.

Hong, H.H., Devereux, T.R., Roycroft, J.H., Boorman, G.A. and Sills, R.C., 1998, Frequency of ras mutations in liver neoplasms from B6C3F1 mice exposed to tetrafluoroethylene for two years, *Toxicol. Pathol.*, **26**, 646–650.

Kocher, O., Cheresh, P., Brown, L.F. and Lee, S.W., 1995, Identification of a novel gene, selectively up-regulated in human carcinomas, using the differential display technique, *Clin. Cancer Res.*, **1**, 1209–1215.

Kullak-Ublick, G.A., Beuers, U., Fahney, C., Hagenbuch, B., Meier, P.J. and Paumgartner, G., 1997, Identification and functional characterization of the promoter region of the human organic anion transporting polypeptide gene, *Hepatology*, **26**, 991–997.

Ledakis, P., Tanimura, H. and Fojo, T., 1998, Limitations of differential display, *Biochem. Biophys. Res. Commun.*, **251**, 653–656.

Liang, P. and Pardee, A.B., 1992, Differential display of eukaryotic messenger RNA by means of the polymerase chain reaction, *Science*, **257**, 967–971.

Madden, S.L., Galella, E.A., Zhu, J., Bertelsen, A.H. and Beaudry, G.A., 1997, SAGE transcript profiles for p53-dependent growth regulation, *Oncogene*, **15**, 1079–1085.

Money, T., Reader, S., Qu, L.J., Dunford, R.P. and Moore, G., 1996, AFLP-based mRNA fingerprinting, *Nucleic Acids Res.*, **24**, 2616–2617.

Murk, A.J., Legler, J., Denison, M.S., Giesy, J.P., van de Guchte, C. and Brouwer, A., 1996, Chemical-activated luciferase gene expression (CALUX): a novel in vitro bioassay for Ah receptor active compounds in sediments and pore water, *Fundam. Appl. Toxicol.*, **33**, 149–160.

Schwahn, D.J. and Medina, D., 1998, p96, a MAPK-related protein, is consistently downregulated during mouse mammary carcinogenesis, *Oncogene*, **17**, 1173–1178.

Shimomura, O., Johnson, R.H. and Saiga, Y., 1962, Extraction, purification and properties of aequorin, a bioluminescent protein from the luminous hydromedusan, Aequorea, *J. Cell. Comp. Physiol.*, **59**, 223–238.

Todd, J., Pachl, C., White, R., Yeghiazarian, T., Johnson, P., Taylor, B. *et al.*, 1995, Performance characteristics for the quantitation of plasma HIV-1 RNA using branched DNA signal amplification technology, *J. Acquir. Immune Defic. Syndr. Hum. Retrovirol.*, **10** (Suppl 2), S35–S44.

Urdea, M.S., 1994, Branched DNA signal amplification, *Biotechnology*, **12**, 926–928.

Vanden Heuvel, J.P., Holden, P., Tugwood, J., Ingle, C., Yen, W., Galjart, N. *et al.*, 1998, Identification of a novel peroxisome proliferator responsive cDNA isolated from rat hepatocytes as the zinc-finger protein ZFP-37, *Toxicol. Appl. Pharmacol.*, **152**, 107–118.

Velculescu, V.E., Zhang, L., Vogelstein, B. and Kinzler, K.W., 1995, Serial analysis of gene expression, *Science*, **270**, 484–487.

Walden, P.D., Lefkowitz, G.K., Ficazzola, M., Gitlin, J. and Lepor, H., 1998, Identification of genes associated with stromal hyperplasia and glandular atrophy of the prostate by mRNA differential display, *Exp. Cell Res.*, **245**, 19–26.

Walsh, A.A., Tullis, K., Rice, R.H. and Denison, M.S., 1996, Identification of a novel cis-acting negative regulatory element affecting expression of the CYP1A1 gene in rat epidermal cells, *J. Biol. Chem.*, **271**, 22746–22753.

Wang, J., Shen, L., Najafi, H., Kolberg, J., Matschinsky, F.M., Urdea, M. *et al.*, 1997, Regulation of insulin preRNA splicing by glucose, *Proc. Natl. Acad. Sci. USA*, **94**, 4360–4365.

Welford, S.M., Gregg, J., Chen, E., Garrison, D., Sorensen, P.H., Denny, C.T. *et al.*, 1998, Detection of differentially expressed genes in primary tumor tissues using representational differences analysis coupled to microarray hybridization, *Nucleic Acids Res.*, **26**, 3059–3065.

Zhang, J.S., Duncan, E.L., Chang, A.C. and Reddel, R.R., 1998, Differential display of mRNA, *Mol. Biotechnol.*, **10**, 155–165.

Zhang, L., Zhou, W., Velculescu, V.E., Kern, S.E., Hruban, R.H., Hamilton, S.R. *et al.*, 1997, Gene expression profiles in normal and cancer cells, *Science*, **276**, 1268–1272.

Note in proof

Dr R. Savory, Roche Discovery, UK

CuraGen

CuraGen Corporation (New Haven, CT) is a company offering gene expression profiling technology based on AFLP. The profiles quantitatively identify differentially expressed genes. Although the technology can be used to analyse samples from any species, knowledge of gene sequences for a given species will facilitate the analysis of gene expression. The technology platform does not require a pre-selection of genes to be analysed, it is an open system.

CuraGen technology is capable of comparing gene expression in two or more samples. The analysis begins with the isolation of mRNA from the samples, which is then converted to cDNA. The cDNAs are digested with a set of restriction enzyme pairs (A and B). The two restriction enzymes cleave each cDNA such that each cDNA yields two to three fragments that have either of the two restriction enzyme sites at the end of each fragment. CuraGen uses a combination of 48 to 96 pairs of restriction enzymes to fragment the cDNA in parallel. They claim that this allows them to cover 95 per cent of all transcripts in the cell. Two-labelled adaptors are selectively ligated to the cDNA fragments using linkers that are complementary to each of the restriction sites (see Figure 4.12). The two adaptors are labelled with either a fluorescent tag or biotin. This ligation step selectively dual labels only cDNA fragments that have both restriction sites at either end of the fragment. cDNA fragments derived from a single restriction enzyme will be labelled at both ends with either the fluorescent tag or biotin.

The cDNA fragments are amplified by PCR using the labelled adaptors (see Figure 4.12). The fluorescently labelled strand from the dual labelled fragment is purified using streptavidin beads. cDNA fragments with no biotin label are not retained by the streptavidin beads. The fluorescent-labelled strand from the dual labelled fragments can then be specifically eluted from the washed beads. This results in the purification of cDNA fragments that are fluorescently labelled and have different restriction enzyme sites at each end of the fragment.

Figure 4.12

Scheme showing the basis for the CuraGen gene expression profiling technology.

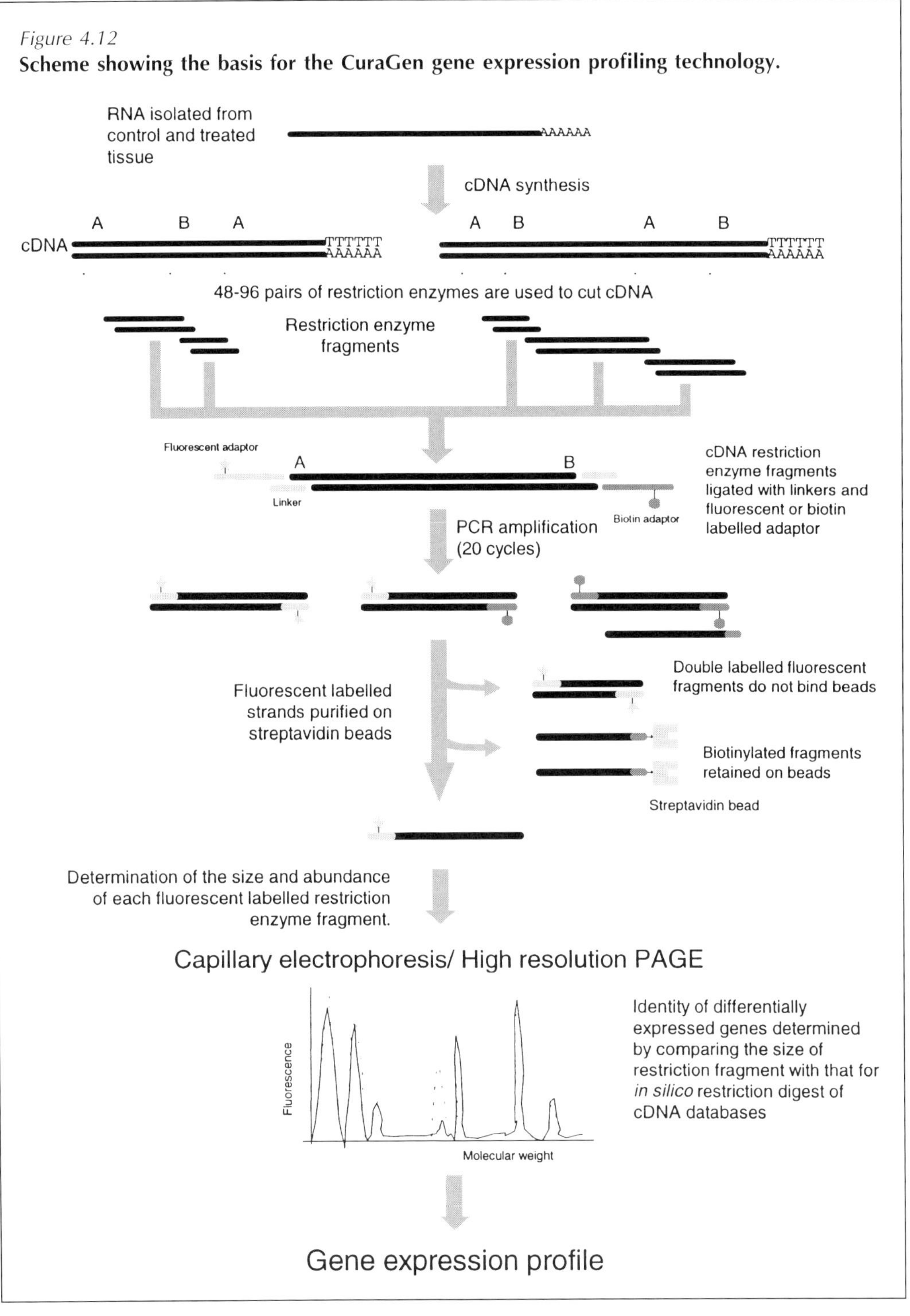

The size and abundance of each purified cDNA fragment is determined by high resolution PAGE or capillary electrophoresis. The abundance of the fragment is proportional to the fluorescent signal as each fragment has only a single fluorescent label. The cDNA fragments that are differentially expressed can be identified and quantified (see Figure 4.12). The fragment size and the sequence information from the restriction enzyme sites are sufficient information to identify the gene giving rise to a specific fragment. To confirm this *in silico* gene identification CuraGen use a technique called 'poisoning'. Poisoning involves repeating the PCR amplification step and replacing the fluorescent adaptor with an unlabelled gene specific adaptor. The pattern of cDNA fragments generated by the poisoned reaction is compared to the original pattern. If the presence of the band in question is ablated in the poisoned reaction the *in silico* gene identification is taken as correct. However if poisoning fails to confirm the identity of a cDNA fragment, or if the differentially expressed fragment is not found in the database, the fragment in question can be isolated, cloned and sequenced in the conventional fashion. The chances of failing to find an *in silico* match for a cDNA fragment is increased in species where there are small sequence databases, such as rat or dog. This is a potential disadvantage with the technology, but as the genomic databases approach closure this problem will become less significant.

5 Early Toxic Stressor Genes – Modulation and Screening Technologies

C.N. Kind and T.G. Hammond, AstraZeneca, UK

5.1 The stress response – a universal but adapted system of cell defence

5.1.1 Cells and the external environment

Since the origin of life, organisms have required the means to protect themselves from hostile external environments in order to survive. Of equal importance in evolutionary terms, development of such protection has enabled successful organisms to endure changing environments and to colonize new ones. Key systems of defence have been retained and elaborated throughout evolution and can be found in prokaryotic and eukaryotic organisms. These include residual protective factors, such as antioxidant and metal chelating molecules, and inducible systems regulated by gene expression (see Figure 5.1). Although highly specialized cells within complex multicellular organisms face a spectrum of stresses similar to that confronting simple single cell organisms (such as agents with a potential to cause oxidative stress or DNA modifications), the extent to which they are exposed to specific stresses will be significantly influenced by their particular function and local tissue environment. Correspondingly, the capacity of specialized cells to protect themselves from these stresses will influence survival. The measurement of a cell's defence response to stress will therefore not only reflect the nature and potency of the stress agent, but also the status and phenotype of the cell itself.

5.1.2 Stress inducible genes

Heat shock proteins (HSPs) are the products of a highly-conserved though structurally diverse group of stress-inducible genes, whose expression is up-regulated in response

Heat shock proteins (HSPs) are the products of a highly-conserved though structurally diverse group of stress-inducible genes, whose expression is up-regulated in response to hyperthermia and a variety of other physical and chemical stresses.

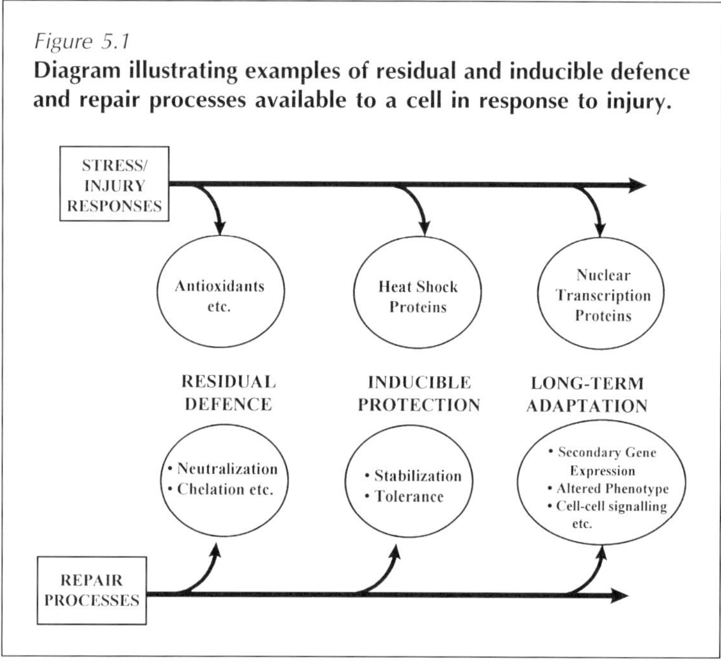

Figure 5.1

Diagram illustrating examples of residual and inducible defence and repair processes available to a cell in response to injury.

to hyperthermia and a variety of other physical and chemical stresses. The effect of thermal shock on chromosomal activity was first described by Ritossa (1962) in experiments using *Drosophila*. This was subsequently linked to changes in expression of a set of specific cellular proteins, initially through work carried out by Tissieres *et al.* (1974). Further characterization of heat-inducible proteins and their closely-related constitutive counterparts has revealed a remarkable series of functionally associated protein families, many of which are involved in essential molecular chaperoning processes in both stressed and non-stressed cells (for a review see Parsell and Lindquist, 1993). A number of HSPs, particularly the molecular chaperones, show distinct subcellular compartmentation according to their function. HSPs resident in cytoplasmic and various organelles, including the mitochondrion and endoplasmic reticulum, work in concert to translocate newly synthesized proteins to their required destination and facilitate their folding into a functionally active conformation (Georgopoulos and Welch, 1993; Stuart *et al.*, 1994). Other HSPs are responsible for the regulation and trafficking of hormone-activated steroid receptors through the cytoplasm into the nucleus (Pratt, 1993). Up-regulation of heat shock protein synthesis following injury provides the cell with an enhanced capacity for the efficient repair or removal of damaged proteins and for processing newly synthesized proteins needed to replace losses (Tomasovic, 1989).

Table 5.1 Major inducible stress protein families

Molecular size/class	Expression in mammalian cells	Intracellular compartment
Hsp 110 kD	Inducible and constitutive	Nucleolus
Hsp 90 kD	Inducible and constitutive Steroid receptor binding	Cytoplasm
Hsp 70 kD	Hsp 72 (inducible) Hsc 73 (constitutive)	Multicompartment
HSP 60 kD	Inducible and constitutive	Mitochondria
Hsp 32 kD (HO-1)	Inducible and constitutive	Not established
Hsp 10 kD	Inducible and constitutive	Mitochondria
Ubiquitin	Inducible and constitutive	Cytoplasm
Grp 78 kD	Inducible and constitutive	Endoplasmic Reticulum
Grp 94 kD	Inducible and constitutive	Endoplasmic Reticulum

These functions are clearly important for survival following injury and many studies have indicated the protective role of HSP induction in tissues such as the heart (Knowlton, 1995), neurones (Lowenstein *et al.*, 1991) and inflammatory cells (Kantengwa *et al.*, 1991).

Historically, HSPs and related proteins have been classified into families according to molecular size. The more widely studied mammalian HSPs are listed in Table 5.1. Proteins comprising the HSP 70 sub-family are among the most highly inducible of the mammalian heat shock proteins. They are also amongst the most highly conserved and show a close homology with a series of proteins in bacteria, yeasts, lower order animals and plants (Nagao *et al.*, 1990). HSP 70 proteins are molecular chaperones and play a central role in the folding, assembly, disassembly and degradation of cellular proteins in both stressed and unstressed conditions (Gething and Sambrook, 1992). Regulation of HSP 70 gene expression has been studied in some detail and work carried out particularly over the last decade has revealed several important components of the underlying control mechanism (Morimoto *et al.*, 1996). A fully detailed picture however, remains to be elucidated. Transcriptional regulation of HSP 70 is established through interaction between Heat Shock Elements (HSEs) located within the promoters of the genes and Heat Shock Factor (HSF) proteins. HSFs are pre-formed proteins located in the cytoplasm and provide an important controlling point for regulation of gene expression

HSFs are pre-formed proteins located in the cytoplasm and provide an important controlling point for regulation of gene expression.

as a result of their reversible inactivation when bound to HSP 70 protein. This provides the cell with a feedback inhibition loop whereby HSP molecules no longer required for stabilization of unfolded proteins are able to down-regulate transcription of the heat shock gene. Conversely, removal of HSP through association with unfolded proteins produced during cell stress allows translocation and trimerization of HSF, with subsequent binding to the HSE. The direct influence of HSP on its own expression presumably enables the synthesis of new HSPs to be efficiently and closely matched to the cell's requirement for protein stabilization, at a time when available metabolic capacity is likely to be compromised and therefore at a premium. Phosphorylation of the HSE-bound HSF trimer is also required for conversion to a transcriptionally active state. Recent work has revealed a modulatory influence of anti-inflammatory drugs on the activation status of the HSF (Amici *et al.*, 1995). These compounds appear to stimulate trimerization and translocation of HSF into the nucleus, thus priming the HSP gene for transcription. Although anti-inflammatory drugs do not by themselves induce DNA expression, their action effectively reduces the threshold for heat shock induction and may relate to the pharmacological properties of this class of compound.

Although HSP 70 family proteins have been studied in greatest detail, numerous other HSPs are stress-inducible and may have useful applications in toxicology. Haem Oxygenase-1 (HO-1, HSP 32) is unusual in that it is induced more strongly by certain classes of chemical than by hyperthermia. Prominent amongst these are oxidizing agents, suggesting a selectivity towards protection against oxidative stress injury (Applegate *et al.*, 1991). This is consistent with the close correlation between HO-1 expression and glutathione status observed in cells (Saunders *et al.*, 1991) and tissue (Ewing *et al.*, 1993). The fact that haem oxygenase is the rate limiting enzyme in conversion of pro-oxidant haemoproteins to antioxidant bile pigments lends support to a functional link between HO-1 and oxidative stress. Moreover, measurement of HO-1 has been proposed as a sensitive method for estimating cellular oxidative stress (Kutty *et al.*, 1994). Haem Oxygenase-1 is not strictly a heat shock protein because of the absence of a HSE within its promoter.

Glucose regulated proteins (GRPs) are a group of molecular chaperones with extensive homology to HSPs. GRP 78 (BiP, immunoglobulin-binding protein) and GRP 94 are particularly associated with the endoplasmic reticulum and possess ER retention signals in the carboxy terminus of their amino acid sequences. These proteins regulate the assembly and trafficking of proteins through the ER system and are constitutively expressed, but are also inducible by glucose deprivation, depletion of intracellular calcium and other stresses (Massa *et al.*, 1996). Other ER resident proteins with chaperone or folding functions include Calreticulin and Calnexin, both of which possess calcium-binding capacity, and HSP 47. GRP 78 and other ER proteins may be involved in the response to ER stress following disruption of calcium homeostasis.

Studies carried out on the constitutive and inducible homologues of HSPs have shown these proteins to have important functions in non-stressed cells. Hence, induction of HSPs can be modulated by a number of other physiological factors in addition to stress. These include determinants of the cell cycle, development and differentiation state, and various growth factors and proto-oncogenes. Accommodation of such diverse regulatory influences is achieved, at least in part, by the existence of multiple forms of HSFs, each subject to differential regulation and activation. Clearly, the effect of physiological modulators on expression of HSPs must be taken into account when these are being used or considered for use as markers or monitors of cell stress.

5.1.3 *Nuclear transcription factors*

Nuclear transcription factors have important regulatory roles in the short and long term initiation and modulation of cellular responses to external stimuli, including those induced by stress. Among the most extensively studied of the inducible transcription factors are the proto-oncogenes c-fos and c-jun (for reviews see Morgan *et al.*, 1991; Hershmann, 1991; Karin, 1997). Stimulation of cell surface receptors through ligand-binding results in activation of c-fos, c-jun and other transcription factor genes via a network of signal transduction pathways and second messengers. The resultant expression of nuclear transcription factor proteins modulates the expression of a plethora of secondary genes. A recently discovered network of signal transduction pathways, the MAPK/SAPK cascade, appears to be specifically responsive to mitogenic signals and stress agents. This cascade utilizes the sequential activation of a series of mitogen-activated protein kinases (MAPK) and stress-activated protein kinases (SAPK, also referred to as Jun-N-terminal kinases, or JNKs) to transduce signals for induction of a number of nuclear transcription factors. These pathways may be

The induction of HSPs can be modulated by a number of other physiological factors in addition to stress. These include determinants of the cell cycle, development and differentiation state, and various growth factors and proto-oncogenes.

Nuclear transcription factors have important regulatory roles in the short and long term initiation and modulation of cellular responses to external stimuli, including those induced by stress.

particularly important in the cellular response to mutagens including regulation of cell proliferation and the development of neoplasia (Simon *et al.*, 1995).

The involvement of c-fos, c-jun and other proto-oncogenes in stimulus-transcription coupling has been demonstrated for both physiological events and pathological processes. In the nervous system for example, long-term potentiation of memory, neuronal development and the response to lesions and chemically-induced seizures have all been shown to involve the induction of c-fos and c-jun (Pennypacker *et al.*, 1995). c-fos, c-jun and related proteins are co-operative transcription factors, forming homo- and hetero-dimeric DNA-binding complexes (AP-1 complexes) with varying DNA-binding activity. Differential expression of c-fos and c-jun can therefore influence the composition of the AP-1 complex, giving rise to the possibility of variation in the resultant secondary gene response (Adcock, 1997). AP-1 DNA binding activity appears also to be redox sensitive and is increased under both pro-oxidant and antioxidant conditions (Schenk *et al.*, 1994), possibly through modification of a conserved cysteine residue in the DNA-binding domain of fos and jun.

The ubiquitous heterodimeric nuclear transcription factor NF-kB possesses DNA-binding activity at many sites on genes of numerous different cell types, but particularly those with involvement in immune responses. NF-kB is activated by a number of agents including a variety of cytokines. Unlike AP-1, NF-kB does not require protein synthesis for transcriptional activity, but is present in the non-stimulated cell sequestrated as an inactive complex with its inhibitory factor, IkB. Activation of NF-kB requires dissociation from IkB and subsequent translocation from the cytoplasm into the nucleus. Redox status is an important factor in activation of NF-kB. Interestingly, cross-coupling between NF-kB and AP-1 appears to result in a synergistic increase in activity at both NF-kB and AP-1 binding sites, thus producing an enhanced response to stimulation (Adcock, 1997).

Apoptosis is a process of programmed cell death vital for the controlled elimination of damaged or unwanted cells. Many toxins can activate apoptosis in cells, although this is often dependent upon the status of the cell and level of exposure to the toxin; higher levels tending to result in necrotic cell death. Conversely, some toxic substances, such as the non-genotoxic carcinogens may suppress apoptotic activity. Unlike necrosis, apoptosis requires the expression of new cellular proteins and a number of genes have been identified as having a role in its promotion or inhibition. In

> Apoptosis is a process of programmed cell death vital for the controlled elimination of damaged or unwanted cells. Many toxins can activate apoptosis in cells, although this is often dependent upon the status of the cell and level of exposure to the toxin; higher levels tending to result in necrotic cell death.

eukaryotic cells, these include c-myc, bcl-2, p53, caspases and fas. Under certain conditions, c-myc together with an associated protein, Max, functions as a transcription factor to drive apoptosis (Green, 1997). This appears to involve activation of ornithine decarboxylase gene expression, which may promote apoptosis through depletion of the intracellular nucleotide pool. Conversely, c-myc expression is markedly increased in response to mitogenic stimuli and in this circumstance may function to promote cell proliferation. Many other genes participate in apoptosis and cell proliferation pathways and it is clear that co-ordinated regulation of these processes is extremely complex, involving subtle, multiple interactions between proteins, and closely regulated gene expression.

The list of genes whose expression is modulated by toxic agents is increasing rapidly, although in many cases their roles are either unknown or not well established. Some of these, including those described above, will undoubtedly provide novel or key information regarding the underlying mechanism of action of specific classes of toxins and may hence become candidate markers for predictive screening against potential toxicity. For example, critical cellular responses to DNA damaging agents are likely to include induction/repression of genes or activation/inhibition of gene products involved in DNA repair, regulation of the cell cycle and apoptotic/cell division decision points. Candidate marker genes here may include p53, WAF-1, GADD proteins.

5.2 Factors that determine the stress gene response

5.2.1 Nature of the noxious agent

The diversity of mechanisms by which chemical and physical agents can adversely affect biological systems has forced organisms to evolve a range of defence strategies to provide effective protection against its external environment. Moreover, induction of gene expression in response to toxic stress and the resultant synthesis of new proteins requires a considerable expenditure of energy by the cell at a time when conservation is of critical importance, as levels may already be severely depleted. Thus, a measured response selectively directed towards specific toxic processes is likely to be the most efficient means by which a cell can initiate an appropriate defence regime and gain maximum benefit from its energy expenditure. It is reasonable to assume therefore that

A measured response selectively directed towards specific toxic processes is likely to be the most efficient means by which a cell can initiate an appropriate defence regime and gain maximum benefit from its energy expenditure.

the profile of genes expressed in response to an injury will be, at least in part, determined by the nature and magnitude of the stress applied. Evidence for selective expression of HSPs has been demonstrated in a number of models (e.g. Jornot *et al.*, 1991). Stress inducers of HSP 72 appear to possess specific characteristics associated with their potential to cause alterations to native proteins (with resultant stimulation of HSP expression through HSF activation, as described earlier). Heat, heavy metals, arsenite and ethanol are all protein denaturing agents and potent inducers of HSP 72. A number of drugs and other chemicals alter cellular proteins by forming adducts as a result of covalent binding, either directly or via metabolic activation. Although there is little information at present to directly link induction of HSP 72 with protein adduct formation, circumstantial evidence for this has been produced for a range of hepatotoxicants (Salminen, 1996) and various other cytotoxic chemicals (Neuhaus-Steinmetz, 1997). Oxidation of protein thiol groups and formation of disulphide-linked aggregates of cellular proteins may also be an important pathway leading to induction of HSP 72 expression (Liu, 1996). Similarly, experiments carried out with acetaminophen and various of its analogues (Bruno *et al.*, 1992), suggests that induction of HSP 32 may be related to the oxidative properties of these compounds.

While altered gene expression induced by early events in the pathogenesis of cell injury may be expected to reflect the mode of action of the toxic agent, genes expressed at later phases, or in response to generalized cytotoxic injury, are less likely to be clearly associated. Furthermore, many physical and chemical agents, such as those with the potential to cause oxidative stress, modulate both stress protein and nuclear transcription factor activated gene expression and these pathways are likely to be closely interrelated, given their respective protective and adaptive roles in cellular responses to injury. A complex pattern of gene expression may therefore result from exposure to a single toxic substance. This will be further influenced by time, extent and frequency of exposure to the toxin.

5.2.2 *Cell phenotype, cell status and tissue-specific factors*

Cells show considerable variation in their response to particular stresses and even cells lines derived from similar origins may exhibit differences in basal (unpublished in-house data) and inducible stress protein expression (Mitani *et al.*, 1990). Responsiveness to stress may be determined

Protective substituents, such as antioxidants, antioxidant enzymes and chelators, constitute a first line defence system in the cell and these, together with other detoxification pathways such as metabolizing enzymes, will tend to attenuate or even eliminate the stress gene response following exposure to a toxic agent.

by a number of cell-dependent factors. Residual levels of protective substituents, such as antioxidants, antioxidant enzymes and chelators, constitute a first line defence system in the cell and these, together with other detoxification pathways such as metabolizing enzymes, will tend to attenuate or even eliminate the stress gene response following exposure to a toxic agent. Induction of gene expression will consequently be subject to a dose-response threshold. Pre-induction of a stress response, using for example sub-lethal heat shock, has itself been shown to attenuate the deleterious effects of a subsequent exposure to heat, or other type of stress (Amin *et al.*, 1995). Although not yet conclusively established, tolerance is probably conferred, at least in part, by the presence of increased levels of the stress proteins themselves. The response time for induction and expression of stress genes is commonly very rapid, occurring within a few hours of stimulation. The half life of the stress gene protein product is generally considerably longer than that of the mRNA transcript and may remain at detectable levels for many days after withdrawal of the stress. Consequently, measurement of either or both mRNA and protein may be necessary in order to determine the dynamics of the stress response. The mRNAs of nuclear transcription factor genes are often targeted for rapid degradation after transcription and their expression may consequently be very transient (Veyrune, 1997). Conversely, gene expression may continue over a protracted period of time when the induction stimulus is maintained. The period over which a regulatory stress gene is expressed will have an important bearing on the way a cell or tissue responds to stress, as for example seen in regenerating liver, where differential expression of the proto-oncogenes c-fos, c-myc and c-jun appear to influence the nature and outcome of the proliferative response to different toxins (Schmiedeberg *et al.*, 1993).

Cell cycle is an important determinant of the stress response. Work carried out by Hang and Fox (1996) showed that heat shock causes HSP 72 and HSC 73 protein to be expressed in a variety of mammalian cell lines in a cell-cycle dependent manner, indicating some form of regulatory mechanism acting upon these genes. Although the authors found no consistent pattern of regulation between the different cell types, it seems likely, bearing in mind their protective role, that HSP induction is an important factor in the differential sensitivity of cells and tissues to stress at different stages of the cell cycle (Westra *et al.*, 1971). Cell phenotype and degree of differentiation also appear to influence the stress response radically. Thus, embryonic astrocytes in culture have been shown to mount a markedly greater stress protein synthesis compared to embryonic cerebral cortical neurones following the same heat shock (Nishimura *et al.*, 1991). The ability of the astrocyte cultures to respond to the applied thermal stress correlates with their greater survival rate, supporting a protective role for these proteins. In contrast to the weak responsiveness of embryonic neuronal cells in culture, fully differentiated neurones produce a vigorous induction of HSPs *in vivo*, when exposed to ischaemic injury (Li *et al.*, 1995), excitotoxic hyperstimulation (Planas *et al.*, 1995) or administration of some NMDA receptor antagonists (Lan *et al.*, 1997). Regional or zonal heterogeneity in expression of HSPs within a tissue may result from differential exposure to the stress agent due for example, to variation in blood supply, or tissue specific factors such as drug metabolizing capacity. The latter is illustrated by the zonal shift in expression of HSP 72 in the mouse liver following administration of cocaine, brought about by prior induction of cytochrome P450 enzymes by phenobarbitol or beta-naphthoflavone (Salminen *et al.*, 1997).

5.3 The utility of stress genes as markers of cell toxicity

The analysis of gene expression, either as specific gene activity or as patterns of multiple gene responses, may have useful practical applications in the study and detection of cell toxicity. In many instances, stress genes display greater sensitivity as markers of early toxic events compared to other more commonly used cytotoxicity endpoints (such as release of intracellular enzymes, cell viability and functional assays). Importantly, early changes in gene expression are likely to relate more closely to the initiating mode of action of the toxic process compared to late stage events, thus providing the possibility for the generation of useful mechanistic data. The subcellular compartmentation and specialized function of some stress proteins may have potential application as organelle-specific markers of toxicity. However, with the possible exception of a few well studied examples, our current understanding of gene responses to toxic agents, their interrelationships with one another and their influence on the resultant cell pathology is very limited. A great deal more information needs to be generated to enable those key stress response genes associated with particular mechanisms of toxicity to be identified. Consequently, the true worth of measuring individual stress genes or gene expression patterns for toxicological evaluation remains to be determined. This is particularly evident with respect to their application to *in vitro* screening systems, where their predictive value for *in vivo* toxicity potential is at present, largely a matter of opinion rather than fact. However, if established as predictive for particular toxicities, *in vitro* screens incorporating gene expression endpoints would have important applications for assessing the toxicity potential of uncharacterized test compounds. Conversely, accumulating evidence for a mechanism-dependent induction of stress gene expression argues against the existence of a 'universal' stress response which could be used as a general marker of all toxic processes.

The usefulness, indeed relevance, of gene expression analysis for prediction of toxicity potential is entirely dependent upon the relevance and applicability of the biological test system employed. In the pharmaceutical industry, the perceived requirement for high volume, rapid throughput screening for selection of lead compounds at an early stage in the development process inevitably means that *in vitro* based systems are the only practical option. However, as already discussed, gene expression responses to potential toxins are critically dependent upon a range of cell and tissue specific factors.

5.4   Detection methods and screening for stress gene expression

Considerable technical advances have been made in recent years that now enable many genes to be studied in parallel and make high throughput screening strategies a realistic prospect. Methods available for the analysis of complex gene expression patterns at the mRNA level include differential display RT-PCR and micro-array nucleic acid hybridization assays. Proteomics technology incorporating two dimensional electrophoresis can be used to determine changes in protein profile.

5.4.1   *Differential display RT-PCR*

This technique enables mRNA species differentially expressed in response to an experimental treatment such as exposure to a potential toxin, to be isolated and subsequently sequenced and identified (if required). The method is limited by the fact that it is not quantitative, possesses an inherent potential for generating false positives and requires subsequent operations to identify selected targets of interest. A further practical limitation is its relatively low sample capacity and requirement for high skill levels.

5.4.2 *DNA micro-arrays*

Nucleic acid probes prepared from cDNA libraries or oligonucleotide sequences and immobilized in fixed arrays onto a solid support can be used to determine the relative abundance of target mRNAs in test and control samples. Arrays can be reduced to micro-scale using glass supports (e.g. Synteni GEM) or silicon chip technologies (e.g. Affymetrix Inc.), enabling the analysis of thousands of genes simultaneously (Lockhart *et al.*, 1996). However, development of micro-array systems requires specialist equipment, necessitating substantial investment of resources. Relatively few manipulations are needed once specimens have been prepared. Currently, DNA micro-arrays have a severely limited sample analysis capacity and are not suitable for high throughput screening.

5.4.3 *Proteomics*

Greatly improved reproducibility together with major developments in protein analysis and data processing capabilities have enabled two dimensional (2-D) electrophoretic systems to be used very effectively for the detection and identification of differentially expressed proteins. By definition, this technique is discriminatory for translated gene expression (unlike mRNA analysis) and is, furthermore, capable of detecting post-translational modifications to expressed proteins. Thus, alterations in phosphorylation state and glycosylation of proteins induced by toxic substances may be detected as shifts in the protein separation pattern. A number of studies have demonstrated the potential for this technique to be applied to toxicology. Time or treatment related changes in the relative tissue concentration of individual proteins can be identified using 2-D electrophoresis, providing useful leads on the mode of action of a toxic compound, as illustrated for example by the down-regulation of calbindin-D in rat kidney following administration of Cyclosporin A (Steiner *et al.*, 1996). Complex changes in protein patterns can also be monitored as, for example, in the development and progression of toxicity over a chronic time course (Cunningham *et al.*, 1995). This analytical approach may be particularly useful for the identification and selection of key patterns of gene expression associated with classes of toxins or lead compounds in drug development programmes. However, its applicability to screening strategies is severely limited by its complexity and relatively slow analytical throughput.

5.4.4 *High throughput screening technologies*

A variety of novel analytical approaches have been devised to facilitate the measurement of *in vitro* gene expression in large numbers of samples. Most of these are based upon cell assays using microplate formats and include systems incorporating the use of reporter gene constructs or mRNA hybridization analysis.

5.4.5 *Reporter gene constructs*

Fusions between reporter genes such as the bacterial CAT gene (Chloramphenicol Acetyl Transferase) and various promoter or response elements of target genes have been constructed and integrated into eukaryotic cells. Commercially available products developed by Xenometrix Inc. include the Cat-Tox Liver assay system (Todd *et al.*, 1995), utilizing modified transformed human liver derived Hep G2 cells containing a battery of stress responsive reporter genes (see Table 5.2a) and the Cat-Tox DNA assay system (Beard *et al.*, 1996), using modified RKO human colon carcinoma cells containing a selection of reporter genes responsive to DNA damage (see Table 5.2b). Both systems adopt a kit format based upon 96-well microtitre assay plates, with quantitative measurement of CAT activity by ELISA. Similar systems developed by Xenometrix utilize genetically engineered strains of *E. coli* with lacZ gene fusions.

Gene expression profiles generated from the Xenometrix assays enable dose response profiles to be constructed, allowing comparisons to be made between test agents (e.g. across a series of structural analogues) or within a therapeutic class of drug. The illustration in Figure 5.2 shows differences between stress gene expression profiles produced in Hep G2 cell constructs in response to cis- or trans- platin. Multiple stress gene responses are seen with the anti-tumour agent cisplatin at 12 µg/ml, whereas the inactive transplatin analogue shows only minimal changes up to 100 µg/ml. Prominent increases induced by cisplatin include the p53 response element, GADD 153 and GADD 45 constructs, indicating a positive correlation between stress gene expression and DNA damaging potency. It is not possible, however,

Table 5.2a Stress gene reporter constructs available in the Xenometrix Cat-Tox Liver assay system

Cat-fusion construct	Description	Inducing agents
CYP1A1	• Cytochrome P450 1A1 • Initiates biotransformation of many chemical carcinogens	• Polycyclic aromatic hydrocarbons • Examples: 3-methylcholanthrene, dioxins, benzo[a]pyrene
XRE	• Xenobiotic response element • Isolated from within the CYP1A1 promoter	• Responds specifically to polycyclic aromatic hydrocarbons
GSTa	• Glutathione S transferase Ya subunit • Catalyzes the conjugation of glutathione to a variety of electrophiles	• Responds to aromatic hydrocarbons and electrophiles (e.g. β-napthoflavone)
HMT IIA	• Metallothionein-II$_A$ • A heavy metal binding protein	• Responds to heavy metals such as arsenic, cadmium, copper, silver, zinc
RARE	• Retinoic response element • Isolated from the retinoic acid receptor beta gene	• Responds to retinoic acid and its analogs
FOS	• c-fos • c-fos is an immediate early gene and proto-oncogene	• Responds to mitogens and some DNA damaging agents
XHF	• Collagenase • Plays a role in the inflammatory reaction	• Responds to mitogens, mitomycin C and UV irradiation as well as IL-1
NFkB	• NFkB response element • Involved in the activation of genes associated with inflammatory, immune and acute phase responses	• Responds to protein synthesis inhibitors, lipopolysaccharides (LPS), cytokines and mitogens
CRE	• Cyclic AMP response element	• Responds to increased levels of cAMP
GADD153	• Growth arrest and DNA damage gene	• Responds to UV irradiation, X-rays, MMS, MNNG and other DNA damaging agents
GADD45	• Growth arrest and DNA damage gene	• Responds to DNA irradiation, X-rays, MMS, MNNG and other DNA damaging agents
p53RE	• Tumour suppressor p53 response element • Involved in the biochemical pathways of cell growth and differentiation	• Responds to DNA damaging agents such as MMS and X-rays
HSP70	• Heat shock protein 70	• Responds to heat, heavy metals, and other protein denaturants
GRP78	• Glucose regulated protein 78	• Responds to increases in intracellular calcium levels and some DNA damaging agents

Table 5.2b Stress gene reporter constructs available in the Xenometrix Cat-Tox DNA assay system

Cat-fusion construct	Description	Inducing agents
βPOL	• DNA polymerase β • Involved in base excision repair	• Induced specifically by agents which cause non-bulky DNA damage
p53RE		See Table 2a
GADD45		See Table 2a
GADD153		See Table 2a
FOS		See Table 2a
TRE	• TPA response element • TRE sites are recognized by the transcription factor AP-1	• Responsive to compounds and conditions which activate protein kinase C
tPA	• Tissue-type plasminogen activator • Cellular protease associated with cellular transformation and tumour promotion • Involved in the cellular inflammatory response	

to directly relate potency of response induced in the cell constructs to *in vivo* potency of the test agent due to the artificial nature of the constructs.

Stress gene constructs using a number of other reporter systems such as luciferase and secreted alkaline phosphatase may confer increased sensitivity of detection to expression assays (Fischbach, 1997). An interesting variant to cell-based reporter assays are those constructed in whole organisms such as nematode worms and *Drosophila* (Welch, 1993). Transgenic strains of the nematode *C. elegans* which produce β-galactosidase as a surrogate stress protein have been used to study the toxicity of various fungicides, and may have useful application in biomonitoring of environmental pollutants (Jones *et al.*, 1996).

Assay systems based upon reporter constructs have the advantage of simplicity and speed of use and are applicable to many different target genes and cell-based test systems. Potential disadvantages largely centre on the artificial nature of the constructs themselves and whether their response characteristics accurately reflect that of the wild type cell. Reporter genes will not detect modulation of stress gene expression at translational level and their products are not functional in feedback control mechanisms as for example with HSP 70 protein (see above). Furthermore, reporter gene products may themselves become significantly cytotoxic if

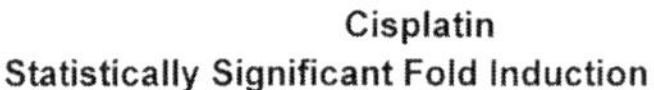

Figure 5.2

3-D histogram representations of the Xenometrix Hep G2 reporter gene construct induction profiles produced in response to (a) Cisplatin and (b) Transplatin exposure.

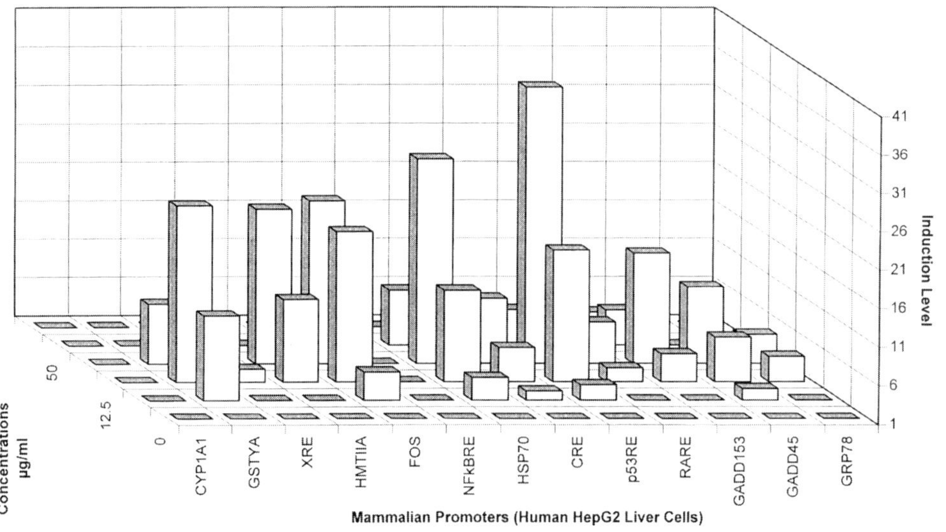

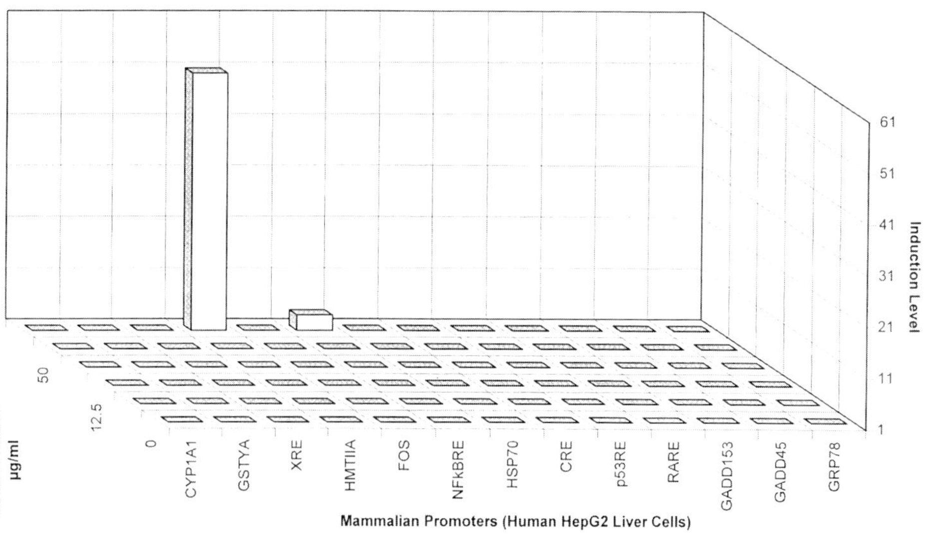

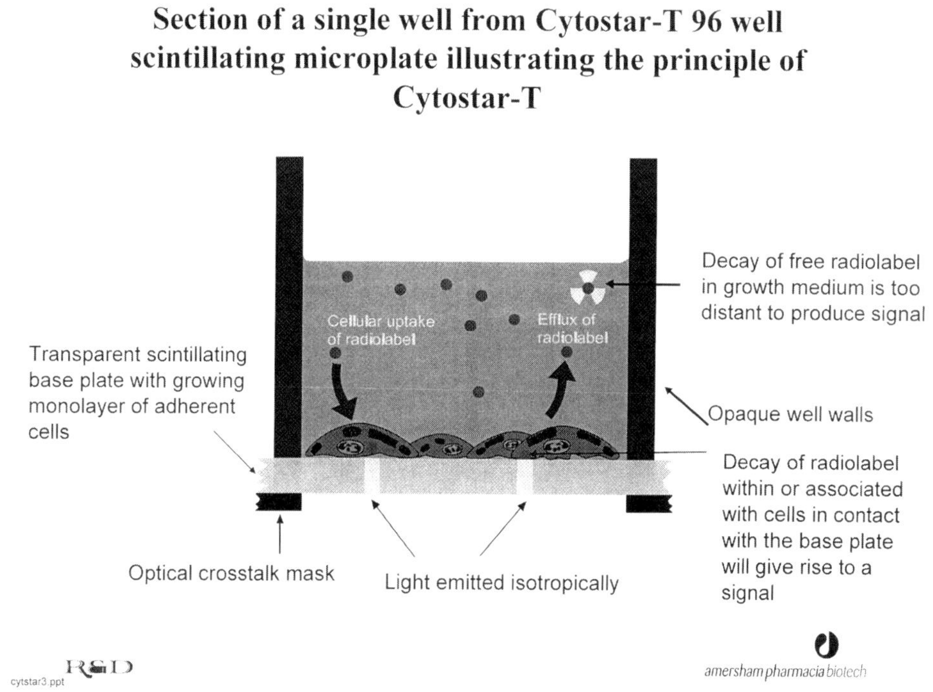

Figure 5.3
Illustration of the concept used in Amersham's Cytostar-T™ scintillating microplate for the measurement of radiolabelled probe. Cytostar-T is a trademark of Amersham Pharmacia Biotech Ltd. © Amersham Pharmacia Biotech UK Ltd 1998 – All rights reserved.

they accumulate to high concentrations. Mammalian cell constructs are at present restricted to the use of cell lines and therefore inherit their limitations with regard to relevance to cells *in vivo*.

5.4.6 *mRNA hybridization assays*

Traditional methods for the measurement of specific mRNA sequences include Northern and Dot- Blot hybridization. Although these methods can produce quantifiable results, they are limited by lack of sensitivity for rare abundance targets, long, time-consuming protocols and low sample capacity. They are consequently unsuitable for high throughput applications. A high volume 96-well plate-based *in situ* hybridization assay, developed by Amersham International plc., utilizes specially designed tissue culture plates containing solid scintillants in a clear base (Cytostar T™ scintillating microplates, see Figure 5.3). Radioisotopically-labelled nucleic acid probes hybridized to mRNA targets in the cell matrix and proximal to the base plate scintillant are detected quantitatively by counting in a suitable instrument. The manufacturer's claim, that 20–30 mRNA copies per cell can be reliably detected by this assay, would enable transcripts of low to medium abundance to be measured, a level of sensitivity compatible with induction of many stress genes. This is supported by work carried out by Harris *et al.* (1996), showing the performance of the Cytostar system to compare favourably with Northern blot analysis, in terms of sensitivity and speed, when used to detect c-fos and G3-PDH (glyceraldehyde-3-phosphate dehydrogenase) in quiescent and stimulated cells. The Cytostar-T assay system can be utilized for monitoring several gene expression profiles in parallel and also in combination with other toxicity endpoints, such as thymidine uptake to indicate cytotoxicity/cytostasis (Swinburne *et al.*, 1997). Although the system is likely to have many applications in work requiring gene expression monitoring, including toxicity evaluation, its reliance on radioisotopic probes for signal detection is likely to limit take-up for HTS purposes.

Quantitative and semi-quantitative gene expression assays based on the amplification of target mRNA by Reverse Transcription-Polymerase Chain Reaction (RT-PCR) represent alternatives to direct detection systems, although at present these have a limited throughput capacity. Assays based on signal amplification techniques, such as the branched DNA (bDNA) concept developed by Chiron (Urdea, 1994), rely on increasing the reporter molecule signal rather than replicating the target and may be more amenable to rapid analysis. Both target and signal amplification technologies are applicable to the analysis of tissues or cells from *in vivo* studies, unlike the Cytostar™ system.

References

Adcock, I.M., 1997, Transcription factors as activators of gene transcription: AP-1 and NF-kB, *Monaldi Arch. Chest Dis.*, **52**, 178–186.

Amici, C., Rossi, A. and Santoro, M.G., 1995, Aspirin enhances thermotolerance in human erythroleukemic cells: an effect associated with the modulation of the heat shock response, *Cancer Research*, **55**, 4452–4457.

Amin, V., Cumming, D.V.E., Coffin, R.S. and Latchman, D.S., 1995, The degree of protection provided to neuronal cells by a pre-conditioning stress correlates with the amount of heat shock protein 70 it induces and not with the similarity of the subsequent stress, *Neurosci. Letters*, **200**, 85–88.

Applegate, L.A., Luscher, P. and Tyrrell, R.M., 1991, Induction of heme oxygenase: a general response to oxidant in cultured mammalian cells, *Cancer Research*, **51**, 974–978.

Beard, S.E., Capaldi, S.R. and Gee, P., 1996, Stress responses to DNA damaging agents in the human colon carcinoma cell line, RKO, *Mutation Res.*, **371**, 1–13.

Bruno, M.K., Cohen, S.D. and Khairallah, E.A., 1992, Selective alterations in the patterns of newly synthesized proteins by acetaminophen and its dimethylated analogues in primary cultures of mouse hepatocytes, *Toxicol. & Appl. Pharmacol.*, **112**, 282–290.

Cunningham, M.L., Pippin, L.L., Anderson, N.L. and Wenk, M.L., 1995, The hepatocarcinogen methapyrilene but not the analog pyrilamine induces sustained hepatocellular replication and protein alterations in F344 rats in a 13-week feed study, *Toxicol. Appl. Pharmacol.*, **131**, 216–223.

Ewing, J.F. and Maines, M.D., 1993, Glutathione depletion induces heme oxygenase-1 (HSP32) mRNA and protein in rat brain, *J. of Neurochemistry*, **60**, 1512–1519.

Fischbach, M., 1997, Stress reporter gene assays for *in vitro* toxicity assessment, presentation at: Cell Culture Models for In Vitro Toxicology, Brescia, Italy 26–31 October 1997.

Georgopoulos, C. and Welch, W.J., 1993, Role of the major heat shock proteins as molecular chaperones, *Annu. Rev. Cell Biol.*, **9**, 601–634.

Gething, M-J. and Sambrook, J., 1992, Protein folding in the cell, *Nature*, **355**, 33–45.

Green, D.R., 1997, A myc-induced apoptosis pathway surfaces, *The Amer. Assoc. for the Adv. Of Sci.*, **278**, 1246–1247.

Hang, H. and Fox M.H., 1996, Level of 70-kDa Heat Shock Protein through the cell cycle in several mammalian cell lines, *Cytometry*, **25**, 367–373.

Harris, D.W., Kenrick, M.K., Pither, R.J., Anson, J.G. and Jones, D.A., 1996, Development of a high-volume *in situ* mRNA hybridization assay for the quantification of gene expression utilizing scintillating microplates, *Analyt. Biochem.*, **243**, 249–256.

Herschman, H.R., 1991, Primary response genes induced by growth factors and tumor promoters, *Annu. Rev. Biochem.*, **60**, 281–319.

Jones, D., Stringham, E.G., Babich, S.L. and Candido, E.P.M., 1996, Transgenic strains of the nematodie *C. elegans* in biomonitoring and toxicology: effects of captan and related compounds on the stress response, *Toxicology*, **109**, 119–127.

Jornot, L., Mirault, M.E. and Junod, A.F., 1991, Differential expression of hsp70 stress proteins in human endothelial cells exposed to heat shock and hydrogen peroxide, *Amer. J. of Respir. Cell & Molec. Biology.*, **5**, 265–275.

Kantengwa, S., Donati, Y.R.A., Clerget, M., Maridonneau-Parini, I., Sinclair, F., Mariéthoz, E. *et al.*, 1991, Heat shock proteins: an autoprotective mechanism for inflammatory cell?, *Seminars in Immunology*, **3**, 49–56.

Karin, M., Liu, Z. and Zandim, E., 1997, AP-1 function and regulation, *Curr. Opin. in Cell Biol.*, **9**, 240–246.

Knowlton, A.A., 1995, The role of heat shock proteins in the heart, *J. Mol. Cell. Cardiol.*, **27**, 121–131.

Kutty, R.K., Kutty, G., Nagineni, C.N., Hooks, J.J., Chader, G.J. and Wiggert, B., 1994, RT-PCR assay for heme oxygenase-1 and heme oxygenase-2: a sensitive method to estimate cellular oxidative damage, *Annals NY Acad. Of Sci.*, **738**, 427–430.

Lan, J.Q., Chen, J., Sharp, F.R., Simon, R.P. and Graham, S.H., 1997, Induction of heat-shock protein (HSP72) in the cingulate and retrosplenial cortex by drugs that antagonize the effects of excitatory amino acids, *Molec. Brain Res.*, **46**, 297–302.

Li, Y., Chopp, M., Zhang, Z.G. and Zhang, R.L., 1995, Expression of glial fibrillary acidic protein in areas of focal cerebral ischemia accompanies neuronal expression of 72-kDa heat shock protein, *J. of the Neurological Sci.*, **128**, 134–142.

Liu, H., Lightfoot, R. and Stevens, J.L., 1996, Activation of heat shock factor by alkylating agents is triggered by glutathione depletion and oxidation of protein thiols, *The Journal of Biological Chemistry*, **271**, 4805–4812.

Lockhart, J., Dong, H., Byrne, M.C., Follettie, M.T., Gallo, M.V., Chee, M.S. *et al.*, 1996, Expression monitoring by hybridization to high-density oligonucleotide arrays, *Nature Biotechnology*, **14**, 1675–1680.

Lowenstein, D.H., Chan, P.A. and Miles, M.F., 1991, The stress protein response in cultured neurons: characterization and evidence for a protective role in excitotoxicity, *Neuron*, **7**, 1053–1060.

Massa, S.M., Swanson, R.A. and Sharp, F.R., 1996, The stress gene response in brain, *Cerebro. and Brain Reviews*, **8**, 95–158.

Mitani, K., Fujita, H., Sassa, S. and Kappas, A., 1990, Activation of heme oxygenase and heat shock protein 70 genes by stress in human hepatoma cells, *Biochem. & Biophys. Res. Commun.*, **166**, 1429–1434.

Morgan, J.I. and Curran, T., 1991, Stimulus-transcription coupling in the nervous system: involvement of the inducible proto-oncogenes *fos* and *jun*, *Annu. Rev. Neurosci.*, **14**, 421–451.

Morimoto, R.I., Kroeger, P.E. and Cotto, J.J., 1996, The transcriptional regulation of heat shock genes: a plethora of heat shock factors and regulatory conditions. In *Stress-inducible Cellular Responses*, Freige, U. (ed), 139–163.

Nagao, R.T., Kimpel, J.A. and Key, J.L., 1990, Molecular and cellular biology of the heat-shock response, *Advances in Genetics*, **28**, 235–274.

Neuhaus-Steinmetz, U. and Rensing, L., 1997, Heat shock protein induction by certain chemical stressors is correlated with their cytotoxicity, lipophilicity and protein-denaturing capacity, *Toxicology*, **123**, 185–196.

Nishimura, R.N., Dwyer, B.E., Vinters, H.V., DeVellis, J. and Coles, R., 1991, Heat shock in cultured neurons and astrocytes: correlation of ultrastructure and heat shock protein synthesis, *Neuropath. & Appl. Neurobiol.*, **17**, 139–147.

Parsell, D.A. and Lindquist, S., 1993, The function of heat-shock proteins in stress tolerance: degradation and reactivation of damaged proteins, *Annu. Rev. Genes*, **27**, 437–496.

Pennypacker, K.R., Hong, J-S. and McMillian, M.K., 1995, Implications of prolonged expression of Fos-related antigens, *TIPS*, **16**, 317–321.

Planas, A.M., Ferrer, I. and Rodriguez-Farré, E., 1995, NMDA receptors mediate heat shock protein induction in the mouse brain following administration of the ibotenic acid analogue AMAA, *Brain Research*, **700**, 289–294.

Pratt, W.B., 1993, The role of heat shock proteins in regulating the function, folding and trafficking of the glucocorticoid receptor, *J. of Biol. Chem.*, **268**, 21455–21458.

Ritossa, F.M., 1962, A new puffing pattern induced by a temperature shock and DNP in Drosophilia, *Experientia*, **18**, 571–573.

Salminen, S.F., Roberts, S.M., Fenn, M. and Voellmy, R., 1997, Heat shock protein induction in murine liver after acute treatment with cocaine, *Hepatology*, **25**, 1147–1153.

Salminen, W.F., Voellmy, R. and Roberts, S.M., 1996, Induction of hsp70 in HepG2 cells in response to hepatotoxicants, *Toxicology and Applied Pharmacology*, **141**, 117–123.

Saunders, E.L., Maines, M.D., Meredith, M.J. and Freeman, M.L., 1991, Enhancement of heme oxygenase-1 synthesis of glutathione depletion in Chinese hamster ovary cells, *Arch. of Biochem. and Biophys.*, **288**, 368–373.

Schenk, H., Klein, M., Erdbrugger, W., Dröge, W. and Schulze-Osthoff, K., 1994, Distinct effects of thioredoxin and antioxidants on the activation of transcription factors NF-kB and AP-1. *Proc. Natl. Acad. Sci, USA*, **91**, 1672–1676.

Schmiedeberg, P., Biempica, L. and Czaja, M.J., 1993, Timing of protooncogene expression varies in toxin-induced liver regeneration, *J. of Cellular Physiology*, **154**, 294–300.

Simon, M.M., Sliutz, G. and Luger, T.A., 1995, Proto-oncogenes and oncogenes in epidermal neoplasia, *Exp. Dermatol.*, **4**, 65–73.

Steiner, S., Wahl, D., Mangold, B.L., Robinson, R., Raymackers, J., Meheus, L. *et al.*, 1996, Induction of the adipose differentiation-related protein in liver of etomoxir-treated rats, *Biochem. Biophys. Res. Commun.*, **218**, 777–782.

Stuart, R.A., Cyr, D.A., Craig, E.A. and Neuport, W., 1994, Mitochondrial molecular chaperones: their role in protein translocation, *TIPS*, **19**, 87–92.

Swinburne, S., Burris, R., Turner, J., Roche, K. and Farr, S. High throughput screening technology, molecular toxicology & bioinformatics: an integrated approach, 1997, 3rd International Conference of the Society of Biomolecular Screening.

Tissieres, A., Mitchell, H.K. and Tracy, U.M., 1974, Protein synthesis in salivary glands of Drosphilia melanogaster: relation to chromosome puffs, *J. of Molec. Biol.*, **84** (3), 389–398.

Todd, M.D., Lee, M.J., Williams, J.L., Nalezny, J.M., Gee, P., Benjamin, M.B. *et al.*, 1995, The CAT-Tox (L) assay: a sensitive and specific measure of stress-induced transcription in transformed human liver cells, *Fund. & Appl. Tox.*, **28**, 118–128.

Tomasovic, S.P., 1989, Functional aspects of the mammalian heat-stress protein response, *Life Chemistry Reports*, **7**, 33–63.

Urdea, M.S., 1994, Branched DNA signal amplification. Does bDNA represent post-PCR amplification technology?, *Biotechnology*, **12**, 926–928.

Veyrune, J.L., Hesketh, J. and Blanchard, J.M., 1997, 3′ Untranslated regions of *c-myc* and *c-fos* mRNAs: multifunctional elements regulating mRNA translation, degradation and subcellular localization, *Prog. In Molec. & SubCell. Biology*, **18**, 35–63.

Welch, J.W., 1993, How cells respond to stress, *Scientific American*, 34–41.

Westra, A. and Dewey, W.C., 1971, Variation in sensitivity to heat shock during the cell-cycle of Chinese hamster cells *in vitro*, *Int. J. Radiat. Biol.*, **19**, 467–477.

6 The Utility of Branched DNA (bDNA) Assays in High Throughput Toxicity Screening

Marque D. Todd, Douglas N. Ludtke, Farshid Oshidari, D. Johnson, and Grushenka H.I. Wolfgang, Chiron Corporation, Emeryville, CA, USA

6.1 Introduction

Monitoring genes which respond to specific types of cellular stress can provide mechanistic information of sub-cytotoxic molecular events.

Early transcriptional responses following exposure to a toxicant are likely to predetermine the later fate of the damaged cell. Genes activated during this early response may include those involved in DNA and protein repair, replication, and growth control. Monitoring genes which respond to specific types of cellular stress can provide mechanistic information of sub-cytotoxic molecular events.

Several technologies exist to detect changes in gene expression from cells or tissues. Common methods include reverse transcription-polymerase chain reaction (RT-PCR), scintillation proximity assay (SPA), and cell lines transfected with promoter–reporter constructs. RT-PCR, a target amplification based strategy, is arguably the most sensitive of all the techniques to measure mRNA levels. However, the technique requires extensive sample preparation and assay optimization, special sample handling areas to prevent contamination, and is at best semi-quantitative. The major advantage of SPA is its homogeneous format which allows for complete automation and increases assay precision. The method proceeds without amplification of the target or signal, thus SPA lacks the sensitivity necessary to detect rare mRNA species. Recombinant cell lines containing promoters of transcriptionally regulated genes fused to reporter genes such as luciferase can also be utilized to monitor changes in gene transcription. This method monitors cumulative gene transcription only, temporal changes cannot be measured.

Because recombinant cell lines are extremely labour intensive to assemble and validate, reporter genes are limited to a few cells types as an indirect assay and may not reflect changes in endogenous gene expression. Other technologies have more recently become available to detect changes in mRNA levels. These include microchip-based assays, fluorescence polarization, and serial analysis of gene expression (SAGE). It remains to be seen if these methods have the required sensitivity and robustness to be used on a routine basis with mRNA.

The Quantigene Assay™ technology utilizes signal amplification to enhance detection of physiologic concentrations of target nucleic acids.

In contrast to many of the methods described above, the Quantigene Assay™ (branched DNA or bDNA) technology utilizes signal amplification to enhance detection of physiologic concentrations of target nucleic acids. In target amplification methods, e.g. PCR, enzymes are used to multiply the number of target nucleic acids available for detection. Because this process involves creating new target molecules, it is subject to the efficiencies/errors of the extraction, purification, and target amplification procedures. With target amplification, reproducible quantification of the original target is not easily achieved. Signal amplification using bDNA technology is based on a series of specific hybridization reactions that are not dependent on complex extraction, purification, or amplification procedures which allows for highly reproducible, quantitative results to be obtained.

bDNA technology can directly measure the level of mRNA transcribed from target genes through a series of specific hybridization events.

bDNA technology can directly measure the level of mRNA transcribed from target genes through a series of specific hybridization events. This methodology has proven to be a highly sensitive, reproducible, and accurate means of quantifying viral load in infectious diseases, specifically human immunodeficiency virus type 1 (HIV-1) RNA (Kern *et al.*, 1996, Pachl *et al.*, 1995, Todd *et al.*, 1995), hepatitis B virus DNA (Hendricks *et al.*, 1995), hepatitis C virus RNA (Davis *et al.*, 1994, Detmer *et al.*, 1996), and cytomegalovirus DNA (Flood *et al.*, 1997). bDNA technology has also been used to study the expression of other intracellular messages. For example, assays have been developed for the direct quantification of human cytokine mRNAs, including tumour necrosis factor-α, interleukin-2, IL-4, IL-6, IL-10, and interferon-γ (Shen *et al.*, 1998).

The bDNA format is flexible which allows experiments to be designed to suit the end user.

6.2   Cell-based bDNA assay

The bDNA format is flexible which allows experiments to be designed to suit the end user. For instance, if cultured cells are used, 96-well plates can be formatted to include a

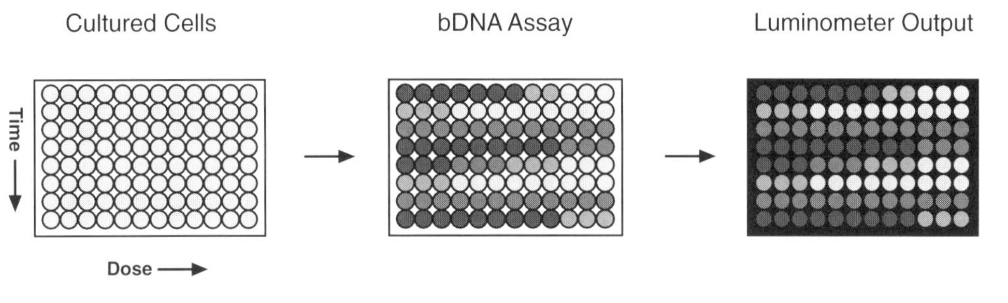

Figure 6.1
Format of cell-based bDNA assay. The cell-based bDNA assay requires two 96-well plates. The first plate is used to culture either primary cells or cells lines. Cells can be exposed to compound in both a time and concentration-dependent fashion. Cells are lysed *in situ* and transferred to a second 96-well plate coated with a capture oligonucleotide where the bDNA assay protocol is performed. The final step of the assay requires reading the light output on a standard luminometer.

range of doses or time points. The general format of the bDNA assay is shown in Figure 6.1. Lysates of cultured cells or tissues can serve as the starting sample. The first step of the assay involves disrupting cells to yield target mRNA that is available for hybridization. This is accomplished by incubating the cells with a lysis buffer containing a detergent, Proteinase K and a gene specific probe set. For cell-based bDNA assays, all manipulations are carried out in a 96-well plate format.

Two distinct sets of target probes are added to the lysis buffer before cellular lysis. The first set of target probes, specified capture extenders, hybridize to the mRNA of interest and to a universal oligonucleotide covalently bound to each microwell of the bDNA assay plate. A second set of probes, known as label extenders, hybridize to areas different from those covered by capture extenders on the target mRNA. The target specific portion of each capture or label extender is approximately 30 bases long. Cellular lysis takes place *in situ* at 55°C for 15 minutes. Lysate (including probes) is transferred to the bDNA assay plate. The hybridization of probes to mRNA and concurrently to the bDNA microwell occurs at 53°C for 16 hours. Since each target molecule is bound to multiple label extenders, signal amplification begins at this step (see Figure 6.2).

A branched DNA oligonucleotide (amplifier) is used to maximize the amount of signal generated from each target mRNA captured on the surface of the microwell. The amplifier hybridizes to the amplifier-specific portion of each

Figure 6.2

Schematic of the bDNA signal amplification assay for mRNA quantification. Similar to an ELISA in its basic approach, the bDNA assay utilizes a solution phase sandwich assay format in which mRNA is hybridized with oligonucleotide probes.

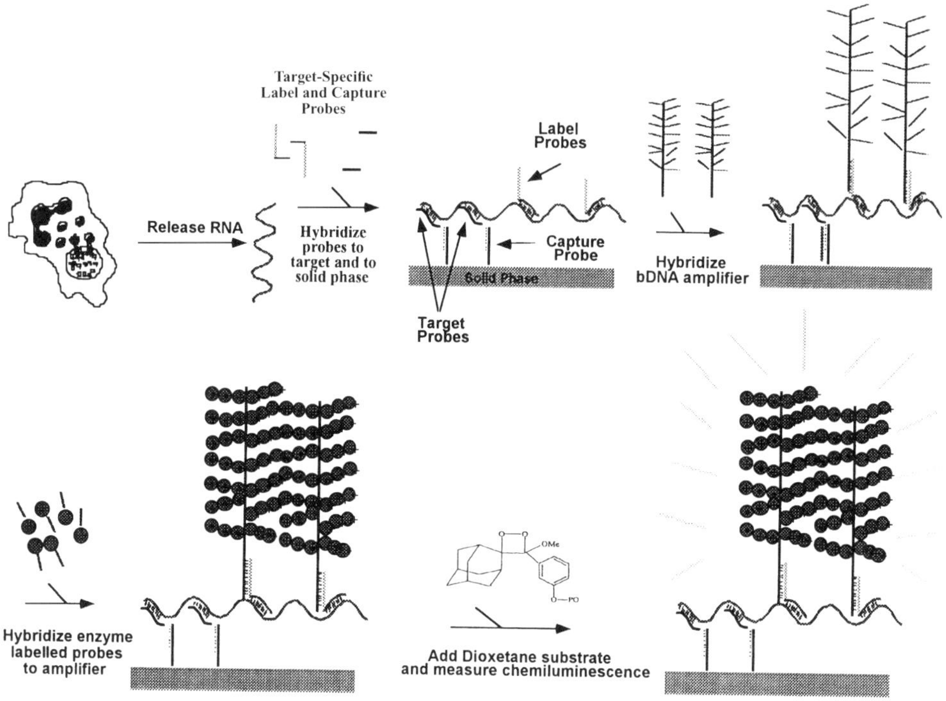

label extender. The cellular lysate is washed from the assay plates and amplifier is added. Amplifier hybridization takes place at 53°C for 30 minutes. Once amplifier molecules have hybridized to the label extenders, the microwells are washed and label probes are added. These probes are short oligonucleotides that have been end-labelled with alkaline phosphatase (Urdea *et al.*, 1988). The sequence of each label probe is complementary to three binding sites on each branch of the amplifier molecule. The amplifier molecule contains 15 branches and each amplifier can theoretically bind up to 45 separate label probes (Horn and Urdea, 1989). Hybridization of label probes occurs at 53°C for 15 minutes.

In the final step of the assay, the labelled amplifier complexes are detected with an alkaline phosphatase triggered dioxetane substrate. Excess label probes are washed from the microwells and substrate is added. The enzymatic conversion of substrate takes place at 37°C for 30 minutes. The chemiluminescent output is read on a 96-well plate luminometer and reported in relative luminescent units (RLUs). The luminometer can be interfaced with a data management system.

Software has been specifically developed to aid in the target selection and probe design process. The software, Probe Designer™, helps to define the target nucleic acid sequence, generate and assign probes, and screen for potential cross hybridization of probe sequences. A variety of options are incorporated into the Probe Designer software. These options include selection of oligonucleotides with constant lengths or constant melting temperatures (Tm). The software also helps develop probes with contiguous sequence alignment, an important part of bDNA probe set development. Using Probe Designer, it can be determined if proposed probe sets can be used to detect the same gene in other species.

The cell-based bDNA assay requires little in the way of specialized laboratory equipment due to its familiar ELISA-style format. Basic tissue culture facilities and liquid handling devices as well as a luminometer is all that is needed to successfully implement the assay in the laboratory. The assay requires approximately one and a half days of total run time with approximately two hours of actual hands-on time. Thus, the assay is easy to implement, requires little labour, and final results can be obtained in as little as 48 hours.

6.3   bDNA assays for toxicity screening

bDNA probe sets have been designed to detect a variety of stress genes. Probe sets for genes that detect changes in response to DNA damaging agents including gadd45 (growth arrest and DNA damage) and gadd153 have been optimized. Probes sets have also been developed for the c-*fos* and HSP70 (heat shock protein) genes. Monitoring genes involved in biotransformation can also be useful for the toxicologist. Probe sets have been designed for human cytochrome P450 3A4 (CYP3A4), rat CYP3A1 and quinone reductase (NQO-1).

The gadd45 protein is found in the nucleus and is transcriptionally regulated throughout the cell cycle being maximal in G_1 (Zhan *et al.*, 1994; Carrier *et al.*, 1994; Smith *et al.*, 1994). It is over-expressed under conditions of growth arrest or DNA damage (Hollander *et al.*, 1993). The N terminus of gadd45 binds PCNA (proliferating cell nuclear antigen), a protein involved in DNA replication and repair. It has been proposed that PCNA–gadd45 interactions may coordinate cell cycle and DNA repair, linking DNA damage responses and cell cycle progression (Hall *et al.*, 1995). The

bDNA probe sets have been designed to detect a variety of stress genes.

gadd153 gene also encodes a nuclear protein and has strong sequence similarity with CAAT enhancer-binding proteins (C/EBP), a family of transcription factors (Ron and Habener, 1992). It has been suggested that gadd153 is a dominant negative inhibitor of C/EBP transcription factors. The relationship between these interactions and the increase in gadd153 expression in response to DNA damage is currently unknown (Luethy and Holbrook, 1992).

The c-*fos* gene encodes a nuclear protein that, when bound to the product of the c-*jun* gene, forms the AP-1 transcriptional complex. AP-1 increases the transcription from a number of cellular promoters, including those involved in such cellular processes as cell proliferation, differentiation, and neuronal function (Setoyama *et al.*, 1986; Angel and Karin, 1981). c-*fos* mRNA is induced during development, differentiation of certain cell types, stimulation by growth factors and mitogens, and in response to cell stress caused by DNA damage (Hollander and Fornace, Jr., 1989; van Delft *et al.*, 1993). HSP70 belongs to a family of protein chaperones whose members facilitate correct folding, transport, and localization of mature proteins (Morimoto *et al.*, 1990). Heat shock proteins also associate with denatured or partially unfolded proteins, protecting them from further denaturation and assisting in their refolding. HSP70 is the best characterized of the heat shock proteins (Milner and Campbell, 1990). The expression of the HSP70 gene is induced by a variety of stimuli, including heat shock, heavy metals, inhibitors of energy metabolism, oxidative stress and stimulation with serum (Liu *et al.*, 1996; Mosser *et al.*, 1998).

The most abundant P450 isozymes in human liver belong to the CYP3A subgene family (Gonzalez, 1992). These enzymes are the second most abundant class of P450 enzymes in rat liver with the CYP2C family being the most abundant. CYP3A enzymes are inducible by numerous drugs such as rifampin, dexamethasone, phenobarbitol, and phenytoin (Murray, 1992). NQO-1 is a Phase II biotransformation enzyme that catalyzes the two-electron reduction of quinones and related compounds (Bayney *et al.*, 1989). Quinone reductase can be induced by a variety of xenobiotics such as planar aromatic compounds, phenolic antioxidants, as well as hydrogen peroxide (Rushmore *et al.*, 1991). One mechanism of induction includes activation of the antioxidant response element (ARE) by reactive oxygen species.

A probe set for GAPDH (glyceraldehyde 3-phosphate dehydrogenase) has also been developed. The assay uses GAPDH mRNA levels to normalize the target gene mRNA measurements from each well (Zhao *et al.*, 1995). This helps to correct for standard sources of variability including the number of cells per well and pipetting errors. Following cellular exposure to a drug or chemical, the bDNA assay is performed and the induction level of the stress gene(s) of interest is determined. Fold induction is expressed relative to the basal mRNA level of the gene when not induced.

Figure 6.3 illustrates the use of the bDNA assay to monitor the up regulation of selected stress genes in response to the hepatotoxin, tacrine, and the nephrotoxin, cisplatin. HepG2 cells were exposed to the drugs and the inductions of HSP70, c-*fos*, and gadd45 were measured. Both time and concentration-response were evaluated in a single bDNA assay. c-*fos* and gadd45 were induced by both drugs in a concentration and time-dependent manner. However, the magnitude of the responses to tacrine was greater, with gene induction occurring at earlier time points (c-*fos*) and larger fold inductions being observed (c-*fos* and gadd45) (Figure 6.3B). HSP70 was not induced by either drug. Thus it is possible, using these limited gene induction profiles, to distinguish by both the magnitude of response and temporal response the effects of two drugs with known toxicities.

Measuring gene induction is one tool that can be used to help define the mechanism by which a compound exerts its toxic effect. The bDNA assay format is particularly well suited for the measurement of stress gene induction, either individually or as profiles of multiple genes. A microtitre-based assay in which cells are grown, exposed to agents, and lysed *in situ*, provides a sensitive and specific means for measuring expression of genes involved in the 'stress response'. The microtitre-based format also lends itself to rapid sample processing with the ultimate goal being automation. Importantly, bDNA methodology quantifies expression of genes in their natural milieu, and can thus be used with a variety of cells or tissues.

6.4   bDNA assay performance

In order to adapt an assay for high throughput screening, it must prove to be robust. Several different parameters need to be assessed when monitoring assay performance. Assay specificity is of paramount importance when different target RNAs are being measured. Other parameters to assess include assay precision, dynamic range, signal to noise ratio, and sensitivity.

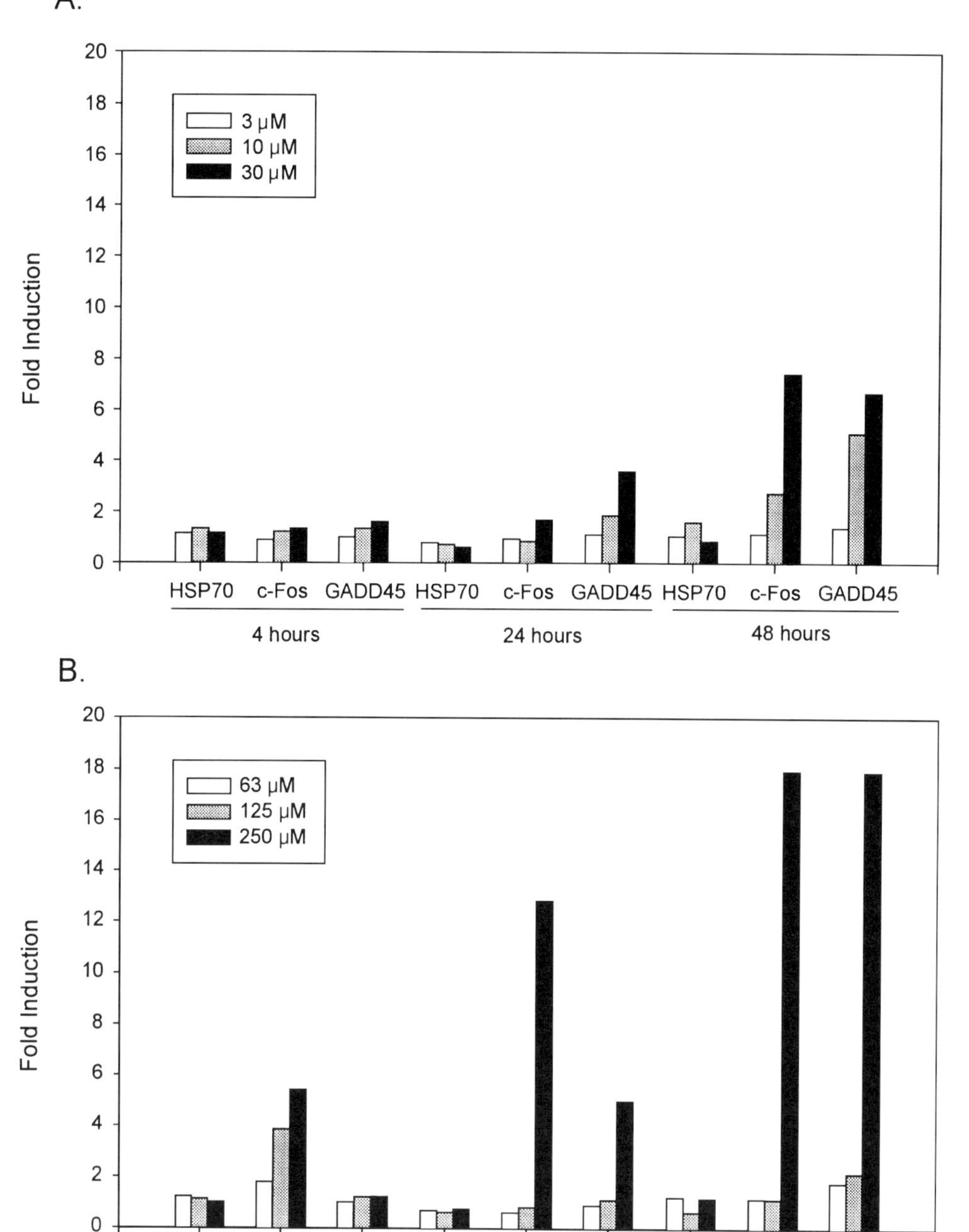

Figure 6.3

Induction of stress genes by cisplatin and tacrine. HepG2 cells were exposed to either cisplatin or tacrine for 4, 24, and 48 hours. Changes in mRNA levels were monitored for the HSP70, c-*fos*, and GADD45 genes. All fold inductions were normalized to GAPDH mRNA levels in cells with a similar treatment. A.) Cells were exposed to concentrations of cisplatin of 3, 10, and 30 µM. B.) Cells were exposed to 63, 125, and 250 µM of tacrine.

6.4.1 *Sensitivity*

The sensitivity, or limit of detection, of Quantigene Assay kits is approximately 7,500 mRNA molecules per sample. It is unlikely that cell-based microtitre assays which measure endogenous mRNA will require greater levels of sensitivity, since approximately 10^4 to 10^5 cells per well are used as the sample input. Even if basal levels of expression of a given gene were only one to two transcripts per cell, several thousand transcripts would be present. This is also true for tissue lysates, given that a 100 mg tissue sample would likely contain over ten million cells.

Generally, the aim is to configure a high throughput assay to give a signal to noise ratio of a least 10:1. The majority of the bDNA assays developed meet this criterion. For example, the gadd45 assay has a ratio anywhere from 20 to 100:1 depending upon the type of cells used in the assay. Similarly, the HSP70 assay can give a ratio between 20 and 400:1. Despite only generating a signal to noise ratio of approximately 5:1, the c-*fos* assay has been used extensively to screen compound libraries. The inherent precision of the fold induction values of this and other bDNA assays ensures that even with relatively low counts meaningful results can be obtained.

At present, assay sensitivity is limited by the background signal. The signal to noise ratio has not been an issue with toxicology probe sets utilized thus far. The background noise of the assay is approximately 2.5 RLU, while the constitutive signal from the least abundant mRNA measured, c-*fos*, ranges from 20 to 100 RLU. The wide range of signal is due to changes in c-*fos* constitutive expression with differences in cellular confluence and diverse cell types.

6.4.2 *Dynamic range*

The dynamic range of the assay can be as important as assay sensitivity. The dynamic range for the bDNA assay configured with the current equipment is approximately three logs. The lower end of the signal range is approximately 2.5 RLU while the maximum linear signal within the linear range is approximately 25,000 RLU. The theoretical dynamic range for the bDNA assay is based upon the background RLUs, signal from the probes without target added, and the upper linear range of the luminometer. All the probe sets designed to date have fallen within four logs, with signal never reaching 25,000 RLU. The amount of signal detected ranges from 20 to 500 RLUs in c-*fos* assays to

Table 6.1 Precision in the cell-based bDNA assay for GADD45 and c-fos mRNA detection

	Raw Data		**Normalized Data**[a]	
GADD45 (6 hr. induction)	Average RLU[b]	Within run RLU CV (%)	Average Fold Induction	Between run Fold Ind. CV (%)
0 μM cisplatin	626.5	6.3	n.a.	n.a.
30 μM cisplatin	1478.2	7.5	2.7	5.2
50 μM cisplatin	1916.8	6.5	3.1	30.1
100 μM cisplatin	1732.0	13.5	3.0	31.2
c-*fos* (6 hr. induction)	Average RLU	Within run RLU CV (%)	Average Fold Induction	Between run Fold Ind. CV (%)
0 μM cisplatin	61.1	28.0	n.a.	n.a.
30 μM cisplatin	164.5	19.0	2.6	0.0
50 μM cisplatin	388.7	12.0	5.8	16.0
100 μM cisplatin	568.2	17.5	10.4	13.0
GAPDH (6 hr. induction)	Average RLU	Within run RLU CV (%)	Average Fold Induction	Between run Fold Ind. CV (%)
0 μM cisplatin	16771.7	4.0	n.a.	n.a.
30 μM cisplatin	16128.7	8.2	n.a.	n.a.
50 μM cisplatin	16337.2	4.9	n.a.	n.a.
100 μM cisplatin	14382.2	10.3	n.a.	n.a.

Two independent runs were performed over an eight week period. Three replicates of each sample were assayed in each run. [a] Fold induction values were calculated by dividing the RLU value for the GADD 45 or c-*fos* sample well by the corresponding GAPDH sample well and then dividing the normalized dosed sample value by the normalized control sample value. [b] Relative Light Units. n.a., calculation of fold induction not applicable.

signals of several thousand of RLUs in the CYP3A4 and GAPDH assays.

6.4.3 *Precision*

Assay precision was evaluated using the gadd45, c-*fos*, and GAPDH bDNA assays. HepG2 cells were dosed with three concentrations of the nephrotoxin cisplatin for 6 hours. bDNA assays were performed and raw RLU values were used to compute within run RLU CVs for the three genes (Table 6.1). Between run fold induction CVs were calculated for gadd45 and c-*fos* after the raw RLUs were normalized to GAPDH (see explanation of calculations in notes for Table 6.1). Within run RLU CVs ranged from 4.0 to 28.0%. The within run RLU CVs were the highest for the c-*fos* assay and lower for the gadd45 and GAPDH bDNA assays. The higher variability in the c-*fos* assay can be attributed to the transcriptional regulation of the c-*fos* gene. c-*fos* levels can be influenced by numerous environmental factors including cellular confluence and growth rate in addition to the primary treatment. Between run raw RLU CVs are not computed because these numbers can be misleading due to variation arising from differences in cell number between wells of the assay. Target gene RLU values were normalized using GAPDH RLU values to limit the effects of cellular confluence. The obtained between run fold induction CVs of 30% or less are reasonable for a quantitative cell-based assay.

As another measure of assay precision, HSP70 and c-*fos* gene expression was analysed using Northern blot analysis and bDNA assays. HepG2 cells were exposed to the DNA damaging agent methyl methanesulfphonate at a concentration of 100 µg/ml for 4 hours. Cells were harvested and total RNA was extracted. In comparison to a 7.5 fold increase of c-*fos* mRNA seen by Northern blotting, the c-*fos* bDNA assay showed an induction ranging from 6.2 to 8 fold in cell lysates (data not shown). All values were normalized to levels of GAPDH. When purified total RNA was used as the target in c-*fos* bDNA assays, the induction ranged from 4.4 to 5.3 fold. Thus, the induction levels observed in the bDNA assay are in good agreement with those derived from the reference method, Northern blot analysis. HSP70 gene induction was also similar when measured by Northern blot analysis or bDNA assays.

6.4.4 *Specificity*

The specificity of different bDNA assays was evaluated by the ability of two bDNA probe sets, CYP3A1 and NQO-1, to specifically bind their respective mRNAs. The rat hepatoma cell line, H4-II-E, was stimulated with various concentrations of β-naphthoflavone (β-NF) or dexamethasone (DEX) for 24 hours. β-NF, a planar aromatic compound, has been shown to be a model inducer of NQO-1 (Rushmore *et al.*, 1991) while DEX, a synthetic glucocorticoid, is a well-known inducer of CYP3A1 (Quattrochi *et al.*, 1995). NQO-1 was specifically induced by β-NF up to approximately four fold while no induction was seen with DEX (Figure 6.4). CYP3A1 showed the reverse induction profile with strong up regulation observed with DEX and no response to β-NF. Interestingly, an almost 1000 fold increase in CYP3A1 message was observed in response to DEX. This level of induction is a consequence of the very low constitutive levels of CYP3A1 mRNA and highlights the type of dynamic range that can be achieved with bDNA assays.

Figure 6.4

Induction of the NQO-1 and CYP3A1 genes by β-NF and DEX in H4-II-E cells. Cells were exposed to either DEX or β-NF for 24 hours. Concentrations of 25, 50, and 100 µM DEX were used while 37.5, 75, and 150 µM concentrations of β-NF were used. All fold induction values were normalized to GAPDH mRNA levels in cells with a similar treatment.

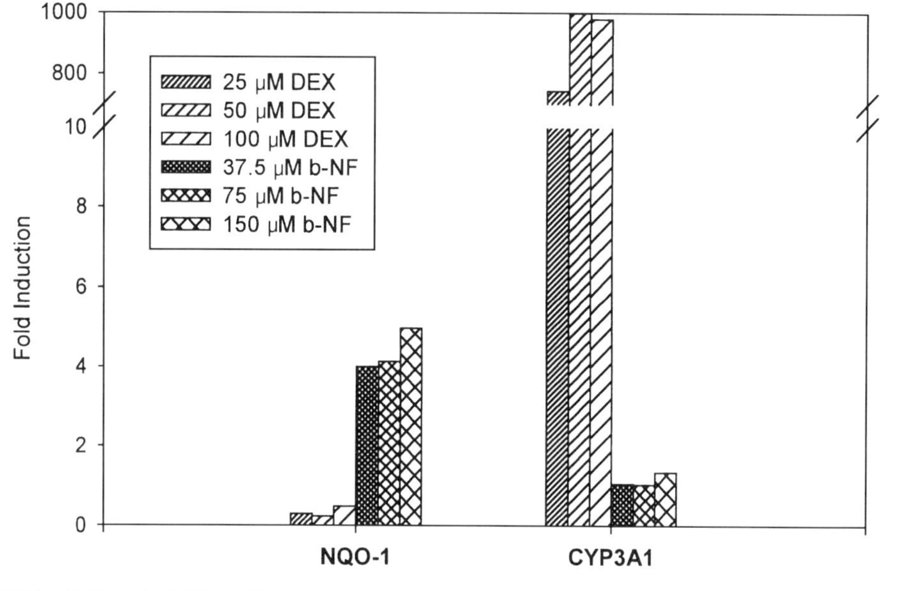

6.5 Automatability of bDNA screening assays

Effective automation is one of the key requirements for high throughput screening. Automation of configured bDNA assays on a variety of robotic systems is relatively straightforward. bDNA screens have already been successfully conducted in a semi-automated format. Some steps of the assay are more amenable to automation than others. For example, the assay requires hybridization to be performed at 53°C after the addition of each new oligonucleotide, yet liquid handling is straight forward. Screens employing bDNA are typically run with volumes ranging between 50 and 300 µl when performed in standard 96-well microtitre plates. The assay utilizes a number of single pipetting steps. Pipetting of these volumes is handled very effectively by the robotic liquid handling instruments currently on the market.

In the semi-automated format, plates are moved manually between pipetting stations and incubators. Throughput for the assay using this format is approximately 20 microtitre plates/day. The move to fully integrate robotic systems with dry and tissue culture incubators will enhance the move towards total automation of bDNA screening assays. This will in turn increase the throughput capacity to at least a 100 plates per day when this technology is chosen for running a high throughput assay.

6.6 Discussion

The ability of bDNA technology to measure the expression of several different genes in both human and rodent cell lines has been demonstrated using known toxicants. Both concentration-dependent and temporal responses were observed. Thus, we have shown that bDNA technology can be used to monitor differences in gene expression in response to different types of toxicants. In addition, we have demonstrated the specificity, sensitivity, and precision of this assay for monitoring changes in mRNA levels.

There are several advantages of using bDNA assays for the measurement of gene induction. Gene expression can be measured directly from cells without the need for recombinant cell lines containing promoter–reporter gene constructs or extraction of RNA. Gene expression can be monitored easily in either cell lines or animal tissues, and RNA from any species can be used with the appropriately designed bDNA probe set. The temporal expression of genes can be measured, enabling the generation of a kinetic profile.

The flexibility of the assay allows for comparisons to be made between many genes to study the mechanisms of toxicity or to screen many compounds and monitor the induction of one gene. As libraries of bDNA probe sets are developed for a variety of target genes, it will be possible to generate gene induction profiles for any given compound. These profiles can be used to rank the toxicity or efficacy of lead compounds or build a structure–activity (or toxicity) database for combinatorial libraries.

Importantly, the 96-well, ELISA-style format of bDNA assays makes them easily automatable and robust enough to be used as high throughput screens. Minimal optimization of individual probe sets and uncomplicated sample preparation greatly enhance the ease of use. Also, contamination is not an issue since the underlying principle of the assays is signal amplification versus target amplification.

The ultimate utility of *in vitro* cell-based assays may be their ability to bridge the gap between *in vitro* and *in vivo* observations. Technologies, such as bDNA, that can readily provide information from cell-based systems, and animals, can be used to develop the necessary correlations to determine the predictive value of gene expression profiles.

The ability of bDNA technology to measure the expression of several different genes in both human and rodent cell lines has been demonstrated using known toxicants.

The 96-well, ELISA-style format of bDNA assays makes them easily automatable and robust enough to be used as high throughput screens.

The ultimate utility of *in vitro* cell-based assays may be their ability to bridge the gap between *in vitro* and *in vivo* observations.

References

Angel, P. and Karin, M., 1981, The role of Jun, Fos and the AP-1 complex in cell-proliferation and transformation, *Biochemica Biophysica Acta*, **1072**, 129–157.

Bayney, R.M., Morton, M.R., Favreau, L.V. and Pickett, C.B., 1989, Rat liver NAD(P)H:quinone reductase, regulation of quinone reductase gene expression by planar aromatic compounds and determination of the exon structure of the quinone reductase structural gene, *Journal of Biological Chemistry*, **264**, 21793–21797.

Carrier, F., Smith, M.L., Bae, I., Kilpatrick, K.E., Lansing, T.J., Chen, C.-Y. *et al.*, 1994, Characterization of human Gadd 45, a p53-regulated protein, *Journal of Biological Chemistry*, **269**, 32672–32677.

Davis, G.L., Lau, J.Y., Urdea, M.S., Neuwald, P.D., Wilber, J.C., Lindsay, K. *et al.*, 1994, Quantitative detection of hepatitis C virus RNA with a solid-phase signal amplification method: definition of optimal conditions for specimen collection and clinical application in interferon-treated patients, *Hepatology*, **19**, 1337–1341.

Detmer, J., Lagier, R., Flynn, J., Zayati, C., Kolberg, J., Collins, M. *et al.*, 1996, Accurate quantification of HCV RNA from all HCV genotypes using branched DNA (bDNA) technology, *Journal of Clinical Microbiology*, **34**, 901–907.

Flood, J., Drew, W.L., Miner, R., Jekic-McMullen, D., Shen, L.-P., Kolberg, J. *et al.*, 1997, Diagnosis of cytomegalovirus (CMV) polyradiculopathy and documentation of in vivo anti-CMV activity in cerebrospinal fluid by using branched DNA signal amplification and antigen assays, *Journal of Infectious Diseases*, **176**, 348–352.

Gonzalez, F.J., 1992, Human cytochromes P450: problems and prospects, *Trends in Pharmaceutical Sciences*, **13**, 346–352.

Hall, P.A., Kearsey, J.M., Coates, P.J., Norman, D.G., Warbrick, E. and Cox, L.S., 1995, Characterization of the interaction between PCNA and Gadd45, *Oncogene*, **10**, 2427–2433.

Hendricks, D.A., Stowe, B.S., Hoo, B.S., Kolberg, J., Irvine, B.S., Neuwald, P.D. *et al.*, 1995, Quantitation of HBV DNA in human serum using a branched DNA (bDNA) signal amplification assay, *American Journal of Clinical Pathology*, **104**, 537–546.

Hollander, M.C. and Fornace, Jr., A.J., 1989, Induction of *fos* RNA by DNA-damaging agents, *Cancer Research*, **49**, 1687–1692.

Hollander, M.C., Alamo, I., Jackman, J., Want, M.G., McBride, O.W. and Fornace, Jr., A.J., 1993, Analysis of the mammalian gadd45 gene and its response to DNA damage, *Journal of Biological Chemistry*, **268**, 24585–24393.

Horn, T. and Urdea, M.S., 1989, Forks and combs and DNA: the synthesis of branched oligodeoxyribonucleotides, *Nucleic Acids Research*, **17**, 6959–6967.

Kern, D., Collins, M., Fultz, T., Detmer, J., Hamren, S., Peterkin, J.J. *et al.*, 1996, An enhanced-sensitivity branched DNA assay for the quantification of human immunodeficiency virus type 1 RNA in plasma, *Journal of Clinical Microbiology*, **34**, 3196–3202.

Liu, H., Lightfoot, R. and Stevens, J.L., 1996, Activation of heat shock factor by alkylating agents is triggered by glutathione depletion and oxidation of protein thiols, *Journal of Biological Chemistry*, **271**, 4805–4812.

Luethy, J.D. and Holbrook, N.J., 1992, Activation of the *gadd* 153 promoter by genotoxic agents: a rapid and specific response to DNA damage, *Cancer Research*, **52**, 5–10.

Milner, C.M. and Campbell, R.D., 1990, Structure and expression of the three MHC-linked HSP70 genes, *Immunogenetics*, **32**, 242–251.

Morimoto, R.I., Tissieres, A., Georgopoulos, C., 1990, Stress proteins in biology and medicine, in R.I. Morimoto, A. Tissieres, and C. Georgopoulos (eds), *Cold Spring Harbor monograph series*, New York: Cold Spring Harbor Press.

Mosser, D.D., Theodorakis, N.G. and Morimoto, R.I., 1988, Coordinate changes in heat shock element-binding activity and HSP70 gene transcription rates in human cells, *Molecular and Cellular Biology*, **8**, 4736–4744.

Murray, M., 1992, P450 enzymes, inhibition mechanisms, genetic regulation and effects of liver disease, *Clinical Pharmacokinetic Concepts*, **23**, 132–146.

Pachl, C., Todd, J.A., Kern, D.G., Sheridan, P.J., Fong, S.-F., Stempien, M. *et al.*, 1995, Rapid and precise quantification of HIV-1 RNA in plasma using a branched DNA (bDNA) signal amplification assay, *Journal of Acquired Immune Deficiency Syndrome and Human Retrovirology*, **8**, 446–454.

Quattrochi, L.C., Mills, A.S., Barwick, J.L., Yockey, C.B. and Guzelian, P.S., 1995, A novel cis-acting element in a liver cytochrome P450 3A confers synergistic induction by glucocorticoids plus antiglucocorticoids, *Journal of Biological Chemistry*, **270**, 28917–28923.

Ron, D. and Habener, J.F., 1992, CHOP, a novel developmentally regulated nuclear protein that dimerizes with the transcription factors C/EBP and LAP and functions as a dominant-negative inhibitor of gene transcription, *Genes and Development*, **6**, 439–453.

Rushmore, T.H., Morton, M.R. and Pickett, C.B., 1991, The antioxidant response element, activation by oxidative stress and identification of the DNA consensus sequence required for functional activity, *Journal of Biological Chemistry*, **266**, 11632–11639.

Setoyama, C., Frunzio, R., Liau, G., Mudryj, M. and De-Crombrugghe, B., 1986, Transcriptional activation encoded by the c-*fos* gene, *Proceedings of the National Academy of Sciences USA*, **83**, 3213–3217.

Shen, L-P., Sheridan, P., Cao, W.W., Dailey, P.J., Salazar-Gonzalez, J.F., Breen, E.C. *et al.*, 1998, Quantification of cytokine mRNA in peripheral blood mononuclear cells using branched DNA (bDNA) technology, *Journal of Immunology Methods*, **215**, 123–134.

Smith, M., Chen, I., Zhan, Q., Bae, I., Chen, C., Gilmer, T. *et al.*, 1994, Interaction of the p53-regulated protein Gadd45 with proliferating cell nuclear antigen, *Science*, **266**, 1376–1379.

Todd, J., Pachl, C., White, R., Yeghiazarian, T., Johnson, P., Taylor, B. *et al.*, 1995, Performance characteristics for the quantitation of plasma HIV-1 RNA using branched DNA signal amplification technology, *Journal Acquired Immune Deficiency Syndrome and Human Retrovirology*, **10** (supplement 2), 35–44.

Urdea, M.S., Warner, B.D., Running, J.A., Stempien, M., Clyne, J. and Horn, T., 1988, A comparison of non-radioisotopic hybridization assay methods using fluorescent, chemiluminescent and enzyme labeled synthetic oligodeoxyribonucleotide probes, *Nucleic Acids Research*, **16**, 4937–4956.

van Delft, S., Coffer, P., Kruijer, W. and van Wijk, R., 1993, c-*Fos* induction by stress can be mediated by the SRE, *Biochemical and Biophysical Research Communications*, **197**, 542–548.

Zhan, Q., Lord, K.A., Alamo, I., Hollander, M.C., Carrier, F., Ron, D. *et al.*, 1994, The gadd and MyD genes define a novel set of mammalian genes encoding acidic proteins that synergistically suppress cell growth, *Molecular and Cellular Biology*, **14**, 2361–2371.

Zhao, J., Araki, N. and Nishimoto, S.K., 1995, Quantitation of matrix Gla protein mRNA by competitive polymerase chain reaction using glyceraldehyde-3-phosphate dehydrogenase as an internal control, *Gene*, **155**, 159–165.

George E.N. Kass and Richard A. Jones, University of Surrey

7 Methods for Assessing Apoptosis

7.1 Introduction

It has been known for over a century that mitosis is an intricate part of the multicellular organization in higher organisms. The first evidence for existence of a physiological and controlled form of cell death dates back to around the same time as a result of the works of Virchow and his students. This form of cell death is an integral component of life as perhaps best illustrated by the loss of the tail structure during the metamorphosis of tadpole to frog. Because a clear spatial and temporal pattern of control of cell death during embryogenesis soon became evident, the term *programmed cell death* was introduced by developmental biologists (Ernst, 1926; Glücksmann, 1951; Lockshin and Williams, 1965; Saunders, 1966). A further milestone in our understanding of cell death was reached when Kerr, Wyllie and Currie coined the term *apoptosis* as they showed that a physiological form of cell death also occurs in the adult animal (Kerr *et al.*, 1972). Since these initial observations, apoptosis has become over the past decade a major focus of research in the fields of biology and medicine. It is now well accepted that apoptosis is a fundamental and ubiquitous process that exists in all cell types in vertebrates (except for mammalian erythrocytes), and that is even found in plants and some unicellular organisms (Kerr *et al.*, 1987; Arends and Wyllie, 1991; Ellis *et al.*, 1991; Jacobson *et al.*, 1997; Rudin and Thompson, 1997).

Although the terms *apoptosis* and *programmed cell death* are often used synonymously, the current consensus is to limit the use of the term *programmed cell death* to the field of developmental biology. This is to avoid the misleading implication that the occurrence of apoptosis is temporally and spatially restricted, and follows a predefined programme. Programmed cell death during development and metamorphosis often occurs with all the features of apoptosis

It is now well accepted that apoptosis is a fundamental and ubiquitous process that exists in all cell types in vertebrates (except for mammalian erythrocytes), and that is even found in plants and some unicellular organisms.

Although the term *apoptosis* and *programmed cell death* are often used synonymously, the current consensus is to limit the use of the term *programmed cell death* to the field of developmental biology.

Table 7.1 Some examples of occurrence and roles of apoptosis

Embryogenesis and Metamorphosis (programmed cell death)
    Removal of excess neurones
    Removal of interdigital webs during limb development
    Regression of tadpole tail (frog)

Tissue homeostasis
    Regression of endometrium, prostate, breast
    Counteract proliferation (liver, intestine)

Defence mechanism
    Killing of mutated and cancerous cells
    Killing of virally infected cells
    Killing autoreactive T lymphocytes

Ageing
    Neutrophils, neurones

described by Kerr, Wyllie and Currie (see below). However, some forms of programmed cell death appear to take place in the absence of those typical features (Schwartz *et al.*, 1993).

Apoptosis dominates the physiological removal of cells during the entire life span of lower and higher organisms (Kerr *et al.*, 1987; Arends and Wyllie, 1991; Ellis *et al.*, 1991; Jacobson *et al.*, 1997; Rudin and Thompson, 1997). As such it forms an integral part of normal tissue homeostatic processes that control the steady state number of cells of an organ, and should be regarded as the natural counterpart to mitosis. Apoptosis is also responsible for the decrease in the size of tissues such as endometrium, breast, liver and kidney in response to alterations in hormonal status or work load (Table 7.1). Another function of apoptosis is the destruction of cells that are potentially harmful to the body. For instance, the removal of cancerous cells, cells harbouring viruses and cells of the immune system that are autoreactive occurs through apoptosis. Failure of apoptosis to eliminate these cells may lead to the development of pathological conditions such as cancer or autoimmune diseases (Table 7.2). In contrast, apoptosis may also directly be responsible for certain diseases when excessively active. Thus, conditions like AIDS, diabetes and neurodegenerative diseases, such as Parkinson's syndrome, Alzheimer's disease and amyotrophic lateral sclerosis, all appear to be caused by an overstimulation of apoptosis (Table 7.2; Thompson, 1995).

Table 7.2   Improper regulation of apoptosis – a major cause of diseases

Examples of diseases involving excessive apoptosis	*Examples of diseases involving insufficient apoptosis*
Infections by viruses AIDS, hepatitis, diabetes	*Cancers* Hormone-dependent cancers (breast cancer, prostate cancer, liver cancer), follicular lymphomas
Neurodegenerative diseases Parkinson's disease, Alzheimer's disease, transmissible spongiform encephalopathies	
	Autoimmune diseases Systemic lupus erythematosus
Immune-mediated diseases Diabetes, primary biliary cirrhosis, thyroiditis	*Infections by viruses* Herpes simplex, infectious mononucleosis

7.2   Apoptosis: morphological features

It is important to remember that apoptosis was initially described by its morphological characteristics, and it is only recently that we have begun to unravel the biochemical events that are responsible for these changes. The general morphological features of apoptosis are summarized in Table 7.3. Although much of apoptosis is a continuum of interlinked events, several early morphological features need to be highlighted. One early change in apoptosis is a shrinkage of the cell. Concomitantly, marked alterations in cell shape occur with the appearance of small protrusions on the cell surface that are commonly referred to as *blebs*, and that yield a budding appearance to the cell (Figure 7.1; Kerr *et al.*, 1987; Arends and Wyllie, 1991). In addition, a striking

Table 7.3a   Morphological features of apoptosis

Early
    Cell shrinkage and detachment from neighbouring cells
    Loss of microvilli and appearance of plasma membrane blebs
    Margination of nuclear chromatin to nuclear envelope
    Organelles (other than nucleus) remain intact

Late
    Nuclear chromatin condensation followed by fragmentation into discrete units (apoptotic bodies)
    Swelling of endoplasmic reticulum and minor changes in mitochondrial morphology
    Loss of blebs and rounding up of cells

Table 7.3b Biochemical features of apoptosis

Early
    Loss of plasma membrane asymmetry and appearance of
    phosphatidylserine on extracellular side
    Expression of novel surface markers
    Proteolysis of cellular constituents
    DNA degradation to high molecular weight fragments

Late
    DNA degradation to oligonucleosomal-length fragments
    Activation of transglutaminase
    Increase in plasma membrane permeability

Figure 7.1
**Morphological changes in Jurkat T lymphocytes undergoing
apoptosis as revealed by phase contrast light microscopy.**
Apoptosis was triggered by activating the Fas death receptor
with a monoclonal antibody. The top photograph (A) shows
control, non-apoptotic cells while in (B) the classical features
of apoptosis (cell shrinkage, plasma membrane blebbing) are
clearly visible after treating cells with anti-Fas antibody for
one hour.

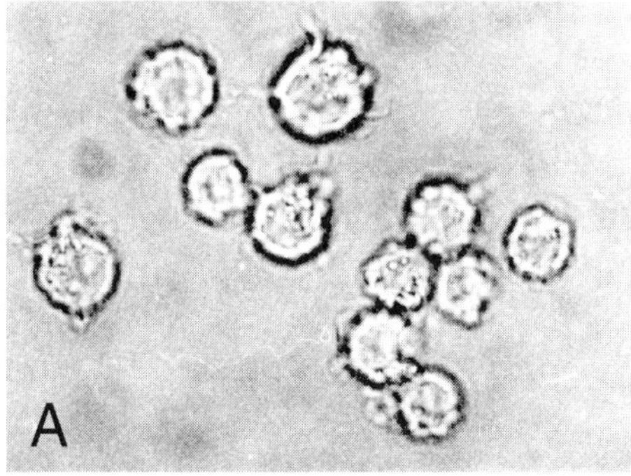

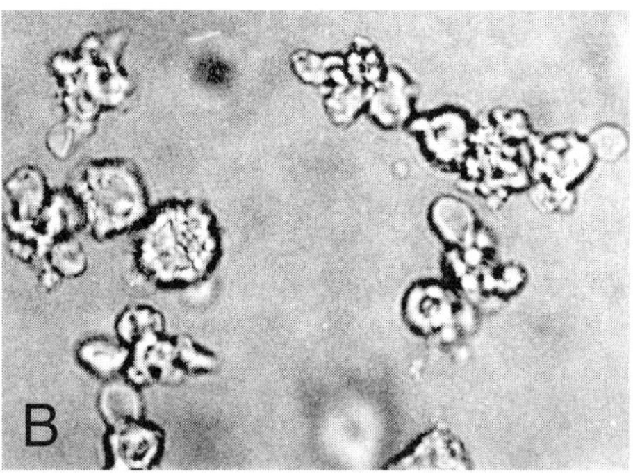

change in nuclear morphology, characterized by a shrinkage of the nucleus and condensation of the nuclear chromatin occurs (Figure 7.2). The normal appearance of the chromatin rapidly disappears in apoptosis as a result of the early margination of the chromatin towards the nuclear envelope and subsequent condensation to produce a doughnut-like appearance. The chromatin further condenses to a concave shape often resembling a half-moon. At this stage the DNA stains strongly with binding dyes giving it hyperfluorescent properties. Subsequently, and as a typically late event in apoptosis, the nuclear envelope breaks up, and the nucleus fragments to form discrete chromatin containing bodies called *apoptotic bodies* (Figure 7.2). In some cell types, such as hepatocytes or Jurkat T lymphocytes, these apoptotic bodies remain scattered within the cell structure stabilized by a rigid plasma membrane (Figure 7.2), whereas cells like thymocytes readily break into discrete units that contain organelles and that are surrounded by the plasma membrane. Electron microscopic analysis of apoptotic cells has shown that most cellular organelles (except the nucleus) initially remain morphologically intact (Kerr *et al.*, 1987; Arends and Wyllie, 1991).

The late morphological changes in apoptosis are not always identifiable *in vivo* because apoptotic cells within an organism are rapidly phagocytosed by macrophages as well as by neighbouring cells. The consequence of this rapid uptake and elimination of apoptotic cells *in vivo* is that the true level of apoptosis occurring in a tissue can be severely underestimated. This is one of the major reasons why the importance of apoptosis in adult tissue homeostasis has remained elusive for so many years.

7.3 Apoptosis: biochemical features

Numerous biochemical and molecular alterations have been described to occur during apoptosis. Early in apoptosis, the nuclear DNA is cleaved into distinct high molecular weight (HMW) fragments corresponding to >700 kilobase pairs (kbp), followed by further degradation to 200–250 and 50 kbp fragments (Figure 7.3; Oberhammer *et al.*, 1993). Finally, these fragments are further degraded to oligonucleosomal-sized DNA fragments that produce a typical ladder appearance when resolved by agarose gel electrophoresis (Figure 7.4; Wyllie, 1980; Arends and Wyllie, 1991). In contrast, mitochondrial DNA remains intact during apoptosis (Murgia *et al.*, 1992). The identity of the endonucleases that cleave DNA is still not

Figure 7.2

Changes in nuclear morphology in apoptotic Jurkat T lymphocytes. Apoptosis was triggered by activating the Fas death receptor using a monoclonal antibody. Aliquots of the cell suspension were fixed and processed for examination by confocal laser scanning microscopy (A,C,E) or transmission electron microscopy (B,D,F). For confocal laser scanning microscopy, the chromatin was visualized by staining its DNA with the fluorescent probe, propidium iodide. The chromatin, which is diffusely distributed in untreated control cells (A,B), rapidly condenses at the nuclear envelope after one hour of treatment with anti-Fas antibody (C,D) followed by the formation of discrete apoptotic bodies after three hours (E,F). Bars correspond to 5 μm (left panel) or 1 μm (right panel).

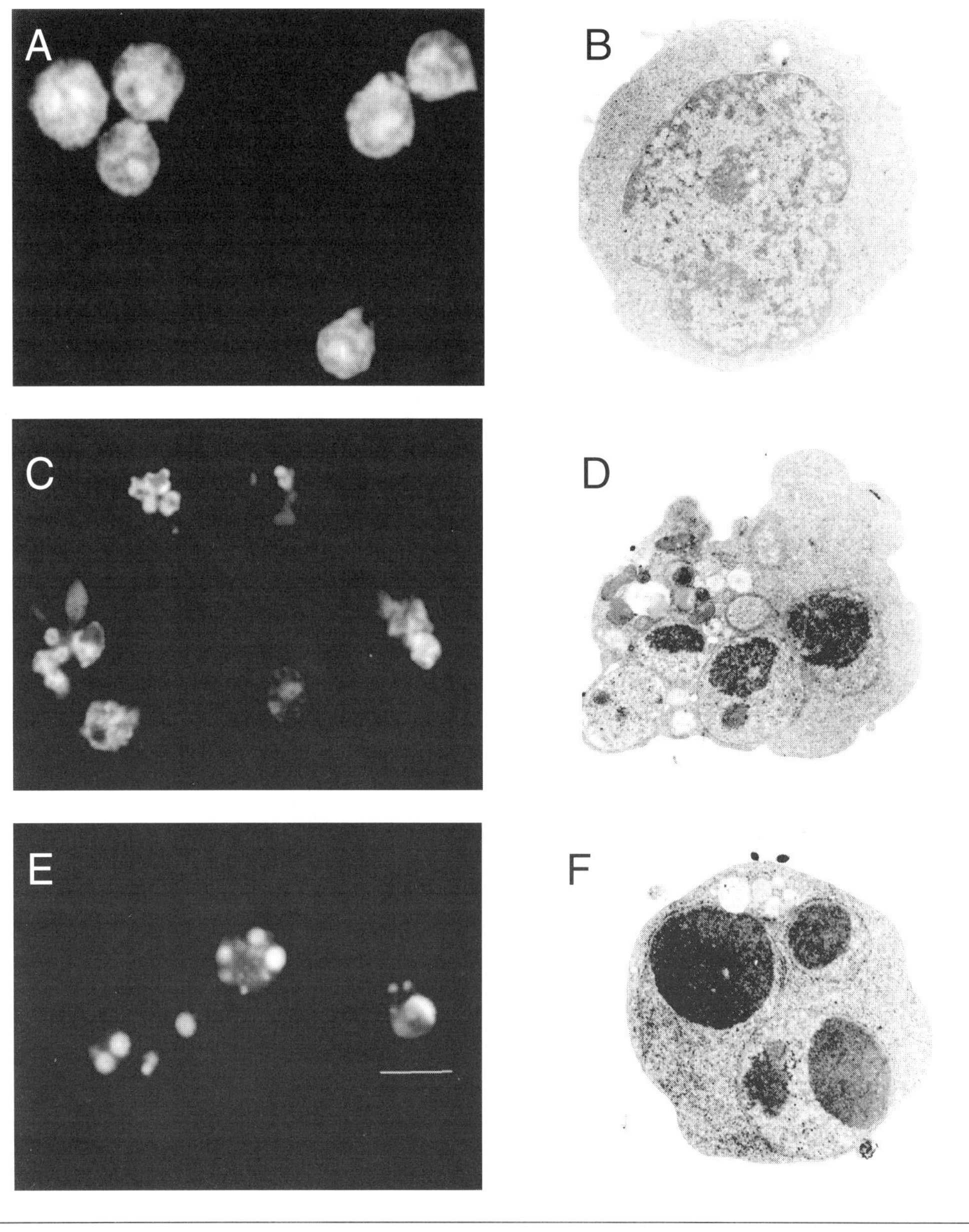

Figure 7.3

DNA degradation during apoptosis as assessed by the formation of high molecular weight fragments. Jurkat cells were treated with anti-Fas antibody and were processed for the examination of high molecular weight DNA fragments by field inversion gel electrophoresis (FIGE). Three major bands corresponding to fragments of sizes >700 kbp, 200–250 kbp and 50 kbp become visible in the apoptotic cells, starting 45 min after anti-Fas antibody treatment.

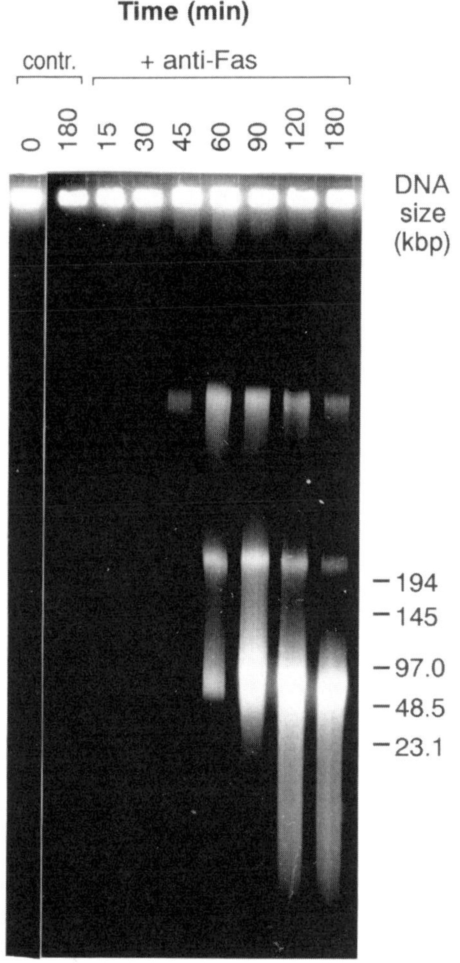

completely established. The formation of HMW fragments is mediated by a Mg^{2+}- and Ca^{2+}-requiring endonuclease (Sun and Cohen, 1994; Zhivotovsky *et al.*, 1994) that appears to be different from the endonuclease(s) that further degrade(s) the fragments to yield nucleosomal- and oligonucleosomal-sized fragments. Numerous endonucleases have been postulated

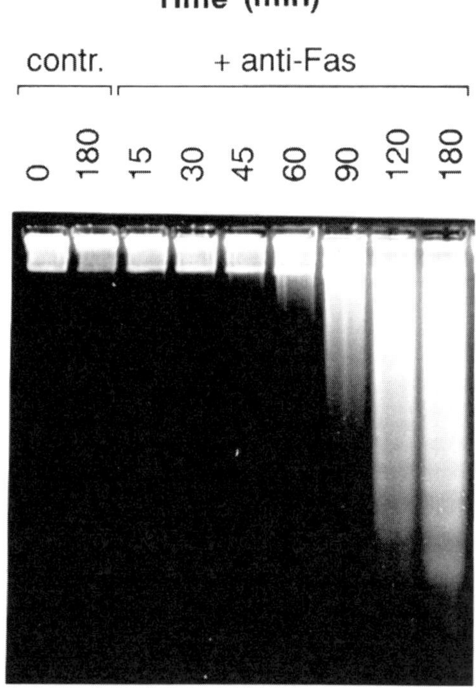

Figure 7.4
DNA degradation during apoptosis as assessed by the formation of oligonucleosomal-length fragments. Jurkat cells were treated with anti-Fas antibody and were processed for the examination of low molecular weight DNA fragments by conventional agarose gel electrophoresis. The degradation of DNA correlates with the appearance of the typical DNA 'ladder'.

to mediate DNA fragmentation in apoptosis, based on their ability to yield a DNA ladder under a range of *in vitro* conditions. Yet, evidence for their involvement in apoptosis has often remained circumstantial. Perhaps more promising is the recent report of an endonuclease referred to as caspase-activated deoxyribonuclease (CAD) or DNA fragmentation factor (DFF) that is constitutively located in the cytosol, where it is found bound to a specific inhibitor (ICAD or DFF45). When ICAD is proteolytically degraded during apoptosis, CAD is freed and enters the nucleus where it will cleave DNA (Enari *et al.*, 1998; Liu *et al.*, 1998).

An additional major characteristic of apoptosis is the activation of a novel family of cysteine proteases that specifically cleave their substrates at a residue that is located next to an Asp residue (at P_1 position). The members of this

> An additional major characteristic of apoptosis is the activation of a novel family of cysteine proteases that specifically cleave their substrates at a residue that is located next to an Asp residue.

family of proteases are called caspases and are related to the prototype enzyme, caspase-1, also known as interleukin-1β converting enzyme (Cohen, 1997; Nicholson and Thornberry, 1997; Villa *et al.*, 1997; Froelich *et al.*, 1998). At least ten different human caspases have been identified, and there is considerable evidence that several of the caspases are responsible for many, if not all, of the features of apoptosis. Thus, the cleavage of cytoskeletal elements such as fodrin, Gas-2, keratins and actin by caspases appears to contribute to the changes in cell morphology. Likewise, the proteolysis of nuclear lamins has been linked to chromatin condensation, and, as mentioned above, the endonuclease thought to cause the degradation of the nuclear DNA requires for its activation the proteolytic removal of an inhibitory factor. One model that is rapidly receiving experimental support is that the caspases are organized in a self-amplifying cascade to allow the rapid and complete execution of apoptosis. The reader is referred to recent reviews (Cohen, 1997; Nicholson and Thornberry, 1997; Villa *et al.*, 1997; Froelich *et al.*, 1998) for a comprehensive discussion on the role of caspases in apoptosis.

Additional biochemical characteristics of apoptosis include the loss of plasma membrane asymmetry with the appearance of phosphatidylserine (PS) on the extracellular side of the plasma membrane (Fadok *et al.*, 1992). The latter event is believed to play a pivotal role in the recognition of apoptotic cells for removal by phagocytosis. Another important event in apoptosis is the activation of the enzyme transglutaminase (Fesus *et al.*, 1987) that cross-links cytoplasmic proteins. This provides a rigid frame structure within apoptotic bodies, and functions to maintain their integrity and prevent the leakage of cellular constituents into the extracellular environment. Finally, there is evidence for changes in sphingolipid metabolism (Hannun, 1996) and calcium homeostasis (Kass and Orrenius, 1999) during apoptosis. How the exposure of PS, activation of transglutaminase and changes in sphingolipid and calcium metabolisms relate to the activation of caspases remains presently unclear.

Research in the field of apoptosis has witnessed a tremendous explosion of activity over the past decade, and our understanding of this phenomenon is now quite substantial.

7.4 Apoptosis: a new challenge for toxicologists

Research in the field of apoptosis has witnessed a tremendous explosion of activity over the past decade, and our understanding of this phenomenon is now quite substantial. Thus, apoptosis can no longer be viewed as an event whose occurrence is spatially and temporally restricted. It occurs following the activation of so-called death receptors, such as Fas (also known as APO-1 or CD95), tumour necrosis factor receptor 1 (TNF-R1), DR-3, DR-4 or DR-5, or the glucocorticoid receptor, as well as in response to the absence of a so-called survival signal (Jacobson *et al.*, 1997; Nagata, 1997; Rudin and Thompson, 1997). Signalling molecules such as interleukin-2, nerve growth factor or epidermal growth factor generate through their receptors signals that are essential for maintaining their target cells alive; in the absence of survival signals these cells die by apoptosis.

Apoptosis can also be triggered by drugs. It is now well established that most (if not all) anticancer drugs that are in current clinical use kill their target cells by apoptosis. This has been observed both *in vitro* (Tomei *et al.*, 1988; Kaufmann, 1989; Walker *et al.*, 1991; Bruno *et al.*, 1992; Zhivotovsky *et al.*, 1993; Ormerod *et al.*, 1994b) and *in vivo* (Gorczyca *et al.*, 1993; Su *et al.*, 1993; Meyn *et al.*, 1994; Meyn *et al.*, 1995; Moreira *et al.*, 1995; Decaudin *et al.*, 1997). The ability of anticancer drugs to induce apoptosis appears to be unrelated to their intracellular target(s). For example, apoptosis occurs in cells exposed to topoisomerase I and II inhibitors (e.g. etoposide, camptothecin), microtubule poisons (e.g. colchicine, taxol) and DNA damaging agents (e.g. adriamycin, cis-platinum, nitrogen mustard, cyclophosphamide).

If most anticancer drugs kill cells by apoptosis, then why are not all cytotoxic chemicals considered as inducers of apoptosis? The reason for this is that most cytotoxic chemicals, when administered *in vivo* or to cells maintained in culture, have traditionally been described to induce cell death by necrosis rather than by apoptosis. Necrosis is viewed as a non-physiological mode of cell death that is fundamentally different from apoptosis (Kerr *et al.*, 1972; Arends and Wyllie, 1991; Majno and Joris, 1995; Trump *et al.*, 1997). Typically in necrosis, the dying cell swells rather than condenses, and substantial damage to intracellular organelles and the plasma membrane are observed. Most compelling is the absence of chromatin condensation and apoptotic body formation. Also, DNA fragmentation, when it occurs in necrosis, is random.

There is little doubt that the rapid loss in cell viability observed when cells are exposed to excessive concentrations of a cytotoxic agent is the result of necrosis. However, under more controlled conditions, the same agents may be capable of inducing apoptosis. For instance, toxic chemicals that generate oxidative stress or induce a pathological increase in cellular calcium levels can kill their target cells by necrosis or by apoptosis, depending on the degree of exposure (Dypbukt *et al.*, 1994; Bonfoco *et al.*, 1995; Raffray and Cohen, 1997). Interestingly, several reports have shown that the product of the anti-apoptotic gene bcl-2 protects cells not only from apoptosis but also from necrosis (Strasser *et al.*, 1991; Kane *et al.*, 1993; Kane *et al.*, 1995; Shimizu *et al.*, 1996). Therefore, the boundaries between apoptosis and necrosis may not be as distinct as often assumed, and it is not susprising that there is intense debate and a large amount of confusion in this area. The nature of the factors that determine whether a cell will die by apoptosis rather than necrosis remains unclear, although current evidence points towards mitochondria. Severe damage to mitochondria, most likely in the form of a permeability transition of the inner mitochondrial membrane (Weis *et al.*, 1994) will result in necrosis rather than apoptosis (Kass *et al.*, 1992; Leist *et al.*, 1997). The link between mitochondria and necrosis could be ATP. Injury that results in necrosis is characterized by a rapid loss in cellular ATP levels (Kass *et al.*, 1992; Rosser and Gores, 1995), and the presence of ATP is required for at least some of the features of apoptosis (Kass *et al.*, 1996; Leist *et al.*, 1997).

An additional complication in the analysis of cell death *in vivo* is that often only post-mortem evidence is available to the investigator. While the features of early apoptosis are generally unmistakable, a late apoptotic cell (if not removed by phagocytosis) will display features of necrosis (in this case often called secondary necrosis) such as swelling of cell and organelles, loss of permeability of the plasma membrane to dyes such as trypan blue or propidium iodide (see below), and finally rupture of the plasma membrane. While it can be argued that late apoptosis may be an artefact of *in vitro* experimentation, it is also clear that when massive apoptosis occurs *in vivo*, proper removal of apoptotic cells fails and massive haemorrhagic and inflammatory tissue damage occurs (Ogasawara *et al.*, 1993; Galle *et al.*, 1995; Kondo *et al.*, 1997). Here, the investigator is faced with histopathology and serum chemistry data that can be very difficult to distinguish from necrosis, in spite of the fact that the form of cell death was apoptosis. Finally, an increasing number of cytotoxic drugs has been found to kill their target cells indirectly through the release of cytokines that act on death receptors rather than through a primary toxic action of the drugs themselves. In the case of the hepatotoxic analgesic paracetamol (acetaminophen), the drug targets both hepatocytes and the resident macrophages called Kupffer cells. The latter respond to the injury by releasing

It is fair to say that with the realization that apoptosis contributes to chemical-induced cytotoxicity, toxicologists are facing novel challenges that will bear consequences on our approaches to the study of mechanisms of injury and risk assessment.

the potent apoptosis-inducing cytokine, tumour necrosis factor α (TNFα), that in turn activates the death receptor TNF-R1 on neighbouring hepatocytes (Blazka *et al.*, 1996; Goldin *et al.*, 1996; Laskin, 1996). In other cases, the cytotoxic drug may induce the expression of Fas ligand in the target cells. This results in the stimulation and activation of Fas and consequently apoptosis of the target cell (Herr *et al.*, 1997). Here also, cell death occurs through stimulation of a receptor rather than through the direct action of the cytotoxic chemical itself.

It is fair to say that with the realization that apoptosis contributes to chemical-induced cytotoxicity, toxicologists are facing novel challenges that will bear consequences on our approaches to the study of mechanisms of injury and risk assessment. In the following sections, we will critically analyse the methods currently available to identify apoptotic cells and discuss their usefulness and reliability in the study of drug-induced cell injury.

7.5 Morphological analysis of apoptotic cells

Apoptosis has been primarily defined in morphological terms, and as such, numerous methods that have been developed to investigate apoptosis are based on specific morphological endpoints. The morphological changes observed in cells dying by apoptosis are unique, and inspection of cells by light or, even better, transmission electron microscopy (TEM) should always be used to confirm biochemical endpoints.

7.5.1 *Cell appearance*

Cells dying by apoptosis undergo dramatic morphological changes. Particularly striking is the shrinkage of the cells that occurs as a very early event during apoptosis and that can be very substantial (up to 30% loss of cell volume) depending on the cell type. The shrinkage of cells is a valuable parameter since it distinguishes apoptosis very clearly from necrosis. For example, cell size is easily assessed by flow cytometry where a decrease in forward light scatter is observed in apoptosis, whereas cell swelling in necrosis is mirrored by an increase in forward light scatter (Telford *et al.*, 1994; Darzynkiewicz *et al.*, 1997). However, as the injury develops and the cells begin to disintegrate, the interpretation of light scattering data becomes problematic.

Plasma membrane bleb formation is easily observed by light and electron microscopy (Figures 7.1 and 7.2). However, blebbing should not be viewed as a phenomenon unique to apoptosis, since it is also one of the characteristics of necrosis, as first documented by Orrenius and co-workers over fifteen years ago (Jewell *et al.*, 1982; Kass *et al.*, 1988; Kass *et al.*, 1992). Although blebs in apoptosis appear different from blebs in necrosis, the difference is often subtle. Particularly with small cells such as lymphocytes, it is difficult to distinguish between apoptosis and necrosis on the basis of the appearance and morphology of plasma membrane blebs.

7.5.2 *Analysis of chromatin condensation*

Chromatin condensation is considered to be a hallmark of apoptosis (Kerr *et al.*, 1987; Arends and Wyllie, 1991), and can be assessed in numerous ways. Most reliable, although fairly time-consuming, remains TEM (Figure 7.2). Alternatively, chromatin condensation can be analysed using dyes that selectively bind to, or become intercalated into DNA (Figure 7.2). These dyes may be used on live or fixed cells or tissue specimens. Some dyes like propidium iodide and ethidium bromide are highly charged and therefore will only gain access to the interior of cells and hence DNA when the integrity of the plasma membrane is compromised. Other DNA-binding dyes, such as the Hoechst fluorochrome HOE 33342 or the new SYTO dyes, freely cross the plasma membrane and their use permits the study of chromatin condensation by fluorometry in living (unfixed) cells.

7.6   Biochemical analysis of apoptosis

Studies into the molecular machinery of apoptosis have sparked an intense search for reliable and, above all, easily identifiable biochemical markers. The pioneering work by Wyllie and co-workers has shown that the condensation of the nuclear chromatin and apoptotic body formation during apoptosis coincide with the degradation of the nuclear DNA to nucleosomal- and oligonucleosomal-length fragments. These appear as a ladder when resolved by agarose gel electrophoresis (Wyllie, 1980). Many of the currently available techniques are based on the detection of cleavage of the nuclear DNA or on the loss of intact cellular DNA during apoptosis. The second group of biochemical endpoints focuses on the changes in the properties of the plasma membrane during apoptosis. Both exposure of PS and alterations in the permeability of the plasma membrane can easily be monitored. Finally, the discovery that proteases, and particular caspases, are the intracellular executioners of apoptosis and that they are responsible for orchestrating most, and perhaps all, changes (biochemical and morphological) reported in apoptotic cells provides us with a range of novel and important biochemical markers for apoptosis. In the following sections we will discuss the advantages and disadvantages of each of these techniques.

It should be noted that a number of additional endpoints have been described in the literature for their potential use in the study of apoptosis. These include changes in mitochondrial transmembrane potential, increases in cytosolic calcium levels and ceramide production and the ability of protein synthesis inhibitors to prevent apoptosis. However, information on the universality of the reported observations (and hence their use as reliable endpoints for apoptosis) is often lacking. More importantly, their specificity for apoptosis over necrosis may be insufficient or even non-existent. This is particularly pertinent to the use of mitochondrial membrane potential and changes in cellular calcium levels as indicators for apoptosis, since both have been known to undergo changes in necrosis as well as in apoptosis (Kass *et al.*, 1992; Kroemer *et al.*, 1997; Kass and Orrenius, 1998).

Commercial companies are competing to develop and market new tests for apoptosis as kits. In many cases, these kits have only been tested on a very limited number of cell lines (raising the question of universality of application). Perhaps of greater concern to toxicologists, these endpoints often suffer from a general lack of information on their ability to discriminate between apoptosis and necrosis. This latter point is extremely important when assessing chemically induced cell death where either apoptosis or necrosis, or even a mixture of the two forms of cell death may occur concomitantly.

7.6.1 *Analysis of DNA fragmentation by agarose gel electrophoresis*

The techniques currently used to assess DNA fragmentation fall into two main categories: the analysis of DNA fragments and the analysis of total cellular DNA content.

The cleavage of DNA into oligonucleosomal-sized fragments is visualized following phenol-chloroform extraction and resolution by agarose gel electrophoresis (Wyllie, 1980). In our laboratory we use the method reported by Sorenson *et al.* (1990) where DNA is liberated from the cells directly into the wells of the agarose gel by *in situ* protease and RNase digestion of the cells prior to electrophoretic separation (Weis *et al.*, 1995). This modification has the advantage of avoiding the solvent phase extraction step and, hence, variations in recovery. Its disadvantage is that in cells with high nuclease activity, such as hepatocytes (Jones *et al.*, 1998), some DNA cleavage by nucleases may occur while the cells are being digested within the wells of the agarose gel. The latter problem can, however, easily be remedied by fixing the cells in 50 per cent ethanol after harvesting to block intrinsic DNase activities (Jones *et al.*, 1998).

In many reports, DNA laddering has been used as the only criterion for apoptosis; yet more recent evidence has shown that in many cell types DNA degradation to oligonucleosomal-length fragments is a relatively late event in the apoptotic process (Brown *et al.*, 1993; Oberhammer *et al.*, 1993; Weis *et al.*, 1995). In some cases, DNA laddering may even be absent despite the obvious morphological appearance of apoptotic nuclei (Cohen *et al.*, 1992; Oberhammer *et al.*, 1993; Ormerod *et al.*, 1994a). The formation of HMW fragments of 300 kbp and 50 kbp correlates more closely to the appearance of apoptotic morphology (Cohen *et al.*, 1992; Brown *et al.*, 1993; Oberhammer *et al.*, 1993; Weis *et al.*, 1995). The nature of HMW DNA fragments remains uncertain. It has been suggested that the 300 kbp fragments represent DNA 'rosettes' made of six chromatin loops of approximately 50 kbp, which become liberated upon further cleavage (Filipski *et al.*, 1990). Internucleosomal cleavage is believed to occur after the formation of the 50 kbp loops.

Given that the appearance of HMW fragments correlates more tightly with apoptosis than does the formation of oligonucleosomal-length fragments, it could be argued that the analysis of HMW fragments should be the preferred approach in the analysis of DNA cleavage during apoptosis. Notwithstanding that the analysis of HMW fragments is very time consuming and requires a technique known as field inversion gel electrophoresis (FIGE), it has recently been reported that HMW fragments are also formed when cells are killed by necrosis (Bicknell and Cohen, 1995). These findings obviously challenge the specificity of FIGE for studying apoptosis. In contrast, it is generally accepted that the presence of a DNA ladder is a reliable indicator for apoptosis, while during necrosis, the DNA is degraded in a random fashion, giving the appearance of a DNA smear when resolved on an agarose gel. However, it is important that gel electrophoresis should not be used as the sole criterion to classify cell death, and above all, the absence of oligonucleosomal fragments should not be used to rule out apoptosis.

7.6.2 In situ *labelling of DNA fragments*

DNA fragmentation during apoptosis is extensive and results in the formation of multiple 3'-hydroxyl (3'-OH) ends. These can be detected by techniques that utilize the ability of enzymes like DNA polymerase or terminal deoxynucleotide transferase (TdT) to add labelled deoxynucleotide triphosphates to the 3'-OH ends of DNA fragments. Most commonly used is a method called TUNEL (TdT-mediated dUTP-biotin nick-end labelling) (Gavrieli *et al.*, 1992). In TUNEL, TdT adds labelled dUTP in a template-independent manner to the 3'-OH ends of single- or double-stranded DNA fragments. TUNEL is therefore a highly sensitive method that can be used to identify apoptosis at the single cell level in cell cultures and fixed or frozen tissue sections. The commonly utilized modified deoxynucleotide triphosphates for indirect labelling are biotinylated dUTP (b-dUTP), digoxygenin labelled dUTP (d-dUTP) and BrdUTP, all of which require a detection system consisting of FITC-avidin or an antibody conjugated to a fluorochrome or enzyme detection system. More recently, single-step TUNEL assays using fluorochromes directly conjugated to deoxynucleotides have been introduced (Li *et al.*, 1995). Detection of apoptotic cells is done by microscopy or flow cytometry.

Overall, TUNEL is extremely sensitive and appears to be highly specific for apoptosis and, therefore, can be considered a biochemical method of choice for identifying this form of cell death. It has been shown that in cells dying by necrosis or when DNA strand breaks were introduced by ionizing radiation or DNA damaging drugs, the number of DNA strand breaks picked up by TUNEL is substantially lower than in apoptotic cells (Gorczyca *et al.*, 1992). However, the universality of these findings needs to be confirmed, especially since it has been known that extensive DNA damage may occur under some necrotic conditions (Ray *et al.*, 1993; Fischer-Nielsen *et al.*, 1995; Dong *et al.*, 1997). An additional drawback of the TUNEL method is that it is only qualitative, i.e. it is not suitable for quantitating the number of DNA strand breaks occurring per nucleus. Modifications have been made to improve the quantitative value of TUNEL but they suffer from a loss of sensitivity (Patel *et al.*, 1995).

> Overall, TUNEL is extremely sensitive and appears to be highly specific for apoptosis and, therefore, can be considered a biochemical method of choice for identifying this form of cell death.

7.6.3 *Immunoassays for the detection of oligonucleosomes*

In addition to agarose gel electrophoresis, a number of biochemical assays have been developed on the basis that nuclear DNA is extensively cleaved during apoptosis. These fragments, which are released from the chromatin during apoptosis (Cohen and Duke, 1984), contain DNA that remains tightly coiled around the core histone proteins. The immunological detection of histones has thus been used as an approach to quantitate apoptosis. The basis of this type of assay is to bind histones of the oligonucleosomes to anti-histone monoclonal antibodies that have been immobilized on a 96-well plate. Using a secondary antibody that is specific for double stranded DNA and that is conjugated to a fluoro-chrome or an enzyme detection system, oligonucleosomes can be detected by fluorometry or an enzyme-linked immuno-sorbant assay (ELISA) (Leist *et al.*, 1994). The selectivity of this technique for apoptosis over necrosis remains to be investigated.

7.6.4 *Measurement of cellular DNA content by flow cytometry*

This approach is based on the selective release and extraction of the low molecular nucleosomal and oligonucleosomal DNA fragments that are formed during apoptosis. The procedure involves the permeabilization of cells with detergents or alcohol fixation, followed by the release by leakage of low molecular weight DNA fragments upon washing of the cells. As a consequence, apoptotic cells are characterized by a lower DNA content. Following staining of the DNA left in the cells with a fluorescent dye such as propidium iodide, SYTO-13 or HOE 33342, the cells are analysed by flow cytometry, and the lower DNA content of apoptotic cells is reflected as a discrete *sub-G_0/G_1* peak of reduced DNA stainability (Ormerod *et al.*, 1992; Afanasyev *et al.*, 1993; Telford *et al.*, 1994; Darzynkiewicz *et al.*, 1997).

The approach based on the measurement of DNA content is rapid and easily performed, assuming that access to a flow cytometer is available. However, a number of variables, including stage of apoptosis, cell type, and DNA extractability, should be borne in mind with this approach. Apoptosis must be confirmed by additional methods since in addition to apoptotic cells, necrotic, damaged cells and cells with a lower DNA content or cells with diminished accessibility to DNA dyes, individual chromosomes and micronuclei will result in an overestimation of apoptosis or even generate false positive results (reviewed in Darzynkiewicz *et al.*, 1997). Likewise, cells not properly fixed may lyse and liberate multiple apoptotic bodies, each of which contributing to the *sub-G_0/G_1* peak, and this will result in an overestimation of the true number of apoptotic cells.

7.6.5 Changes in the permeability properties of the plasma membrane during apoptosis

One of the major distinctions between dead and living cells is that the plasma membrane of dead cells has lost its barrier function between the intracellular and extracellular environments. This is reflected by a reduced ability of dying and dead cells to exclude charged dyes like trypan blue, propidium iodide or ethidium bromide. Likewise, charged dyes that require artificial introduction into cells by an ester loading technique or through microinjection are released from dying and dead cells. Studies into mechanisms of cell death can make use of such dyes to assay the intactness of the plasma membrane. Necrotic and late apoptotic cells have a damaged plasma membrane, and the dyes trypan blue and propidium iodide readily stain cellular proteins and DNA, respectively, whereas these dyes will not in the case of live and early apoptotic cells (Kass *et al.*, 1988; Kass *et al.*, 1992; Weis *et al.*, 1995). As apoptosis progresses, subtle changes in membrane permeability occur and an increase in dye uptake becomes apparent (Ormerod *et al.*, 1993). These changes during early apoptosis are relatively small and are therefore best assayed by flow cytometry.

Other dyes commonly used in apoptosis research, for example HOE 33342 and SYTO-13, diffuse freely across membranes, and accumulate in all cells. Thus, the judicious combination of membrane permeable and impermeable fluorochromes with different excitation/emission spectra can be conveniently used to distinguish between living, apoptotic, necrotic and late apoptotic (secondary necrotic) cells. For example, in a cell population incubated with a mixture of propidium iodide (red fluorescence) and SYTO-13 (green fluorescence), cells will show either green fluorescence or yellow fluorescence (yellow = green + red fluorescence). The cells with green fluorescent nuclei represent live or early apoptotic cells, whereas those with yellow fluorescent nuclei have a damaged plasma membrane and are, therefore, necrotic or late apoptotic. The presence condensed and hyperfluorescent chromatin will reveal the cells that are undergoing apoptosis and differentiate them from live and necrotic cells. Such an approach has been successfully used to elucidate the contribution of necrosis and apoptosis to the death of cerebellar granule cell neurones exposed to the neurotoxic excitatory amino acid glutamate (Ankarcrona *et al.*, 1995).

7.6.6 *Exposure of PS during apoptosis*

Another feature of apoptosis is the loss of plasma membrane asymmetry with the appearance of PS on the extracellular side of the plasma membrane (Fadok *et al.*, 1992). The protein annexin V binds in a Ca^{2+}-dependent manner to negatively charged phospholipids, in particular to PS (Andree *et al.*, 1990). By conjugating annexin V to a fluorochrome such as fluorescein, this property can be utilized to measure apoptosis by flow cytometry (Koopman *et al.*, 1994) or fluorescence microscopy. The binding of annexin V is dependent on its accessibility to PS. Therefore, generalized membrane damage, such as that observed during necrosis or during late apoptosis, will also result in an increase in annexin V binding. This problem of distinguishing between apoptosis and necrosis is easily circumvented by combining annexin V with PI, and experimentally three populations of cells can be distinguished, namely annexin V and PI negative cells (viable, non-apoptotic), annexin V positive and PI negative cells (early apoptotic) and annexin V and PI positive (late apoptotic and/or necrotic) (Figure 7.5). Annexin V and PI combination staining is therefore a technique of choice for studying cell death and should be readily adaptable for rapid screening. The drawbacks of the annexin V and PI approach include the necessity of working with unfixed cells, the critical requirements of Ca^{2+} for annexin V binding throughout the experimental procedure and the necessity to avoid the use of trypsin when harvesting cells (trypsin promotes PS exposure).

7.6.7 *Caspase activation as a quantitative and qualitative measure for apoptosis*

Recent progress has provided us with a number of potential methods to assay for apoptosis that are based on detecting the activation of caspases.

The search for the mechanisms responsible for the features of apoptotic cell death has led to the identification of a family of cysteine proteases called caspases (Cohen, 1997; Nicholson and Thornberry, 1997; Villa *et al.*, 1997; Froelich *et al.*, 1998) that appear to be the key executioners of cell death. Recent progress has provided us with a number of potential methods to assay for apoptosis that are based on detecting the activation of caspases. Two

Figure 7.5

Exposure of phosphatidyl serine during apoptosis. Control and apoptotic hepatocytes were incubated with Alexa™-labelled annexin V and propidium iodide (PI). Panels A and B represent control and apoptotic hepatocytes, respectively, as analysed by flow cytometry. The cells in the middle portion of the graph are negative for both Alexa™ and PI staining and are, therefore, alive and non-apoptotic. The hepatocytes in the upper left corner are positive for Alexa™ but negative for PI staining, i.e. apoptotic. Finally, some cells are found in the upper right corner, and these are positive for both dyes and, hence, considered to be necrotic.

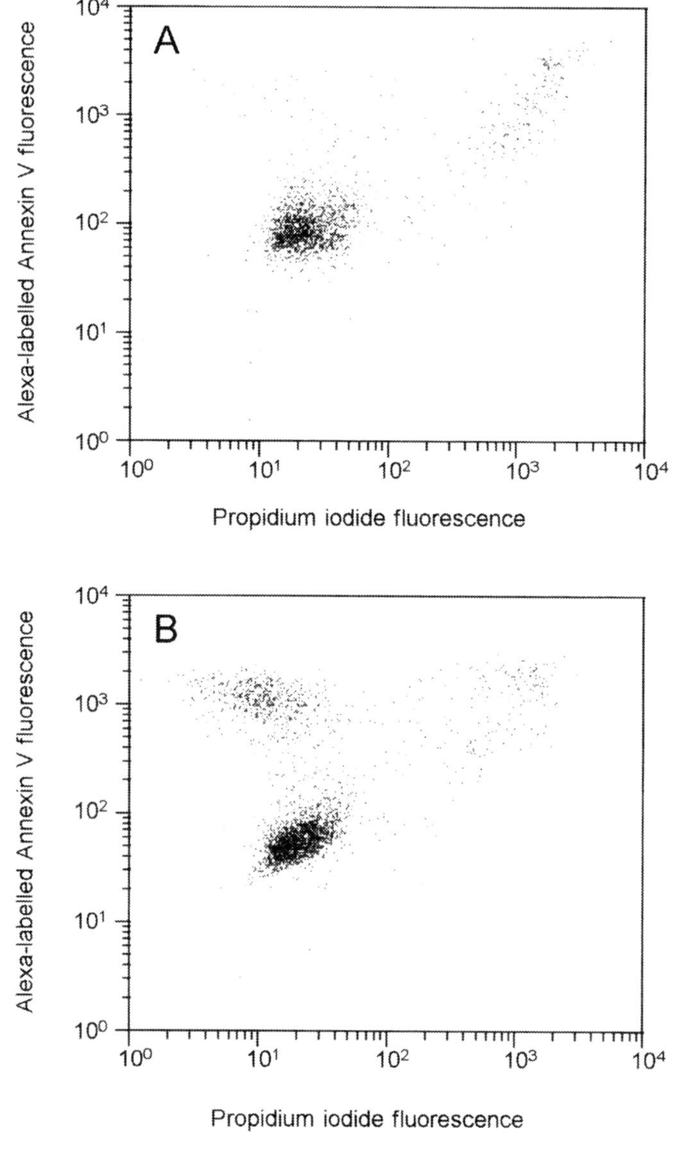

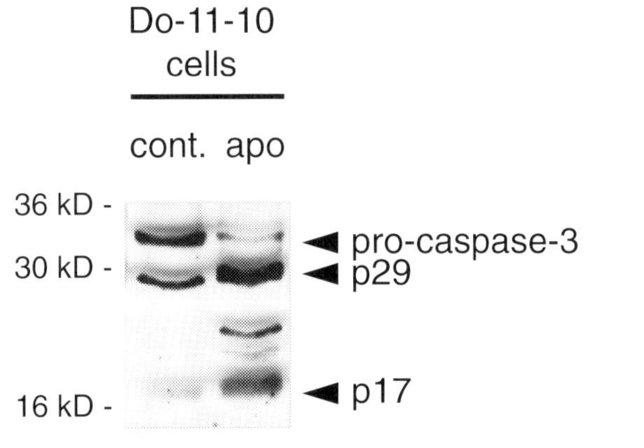

Figure 7.6
Processing of caspases in apoptosis. Mouse Do-11-10 T cell hybridomas were analysed by SDS-polyacrylamide gel electrophoresis followed by immunoblotting with an antibody directed against caspase-3. The effect of triggering apoptosis by exposure of the cells to phorbol 12-myristate 13-acetate and thapsigargin for 20 h is shown by the disappearance of pro-caspase-3 and the appearance of the active fragment, p17.

approaches have been developed, one involving the detection of activated caspases by Western blot analysis and the second approach involving the assay of proteolytic activity, either *in situ* or towards synthetic oligopeptide substrates. Numerous companies are offering antibodies to most currently identified caspases. Under resting conditions caspases are found in cells as inactive proforms, and their activation involves the proteolytic removal of the pro-domain and their further cleavage to a large and small subunit, respectively. Consequently, the activation of caspases is readily assayed by immunodetection of one of the subunits. As shown in Figure 7.6, caspase-3, one of the key caspases in apoptosis exists in non-apoptotic murine hybridoma cells as a 32 kDa pro-form. Upon induction of apoptosis in these cells, the pro-domain is removed and a 29 kDa protein is detected. This form is then rapidly cleaved to the two active forms of caspase-3, p17 and p12, of which the detection of p17 is shown here. This experimental approach is, however, relatively novel since antibodies have only recently become commercially available. Also the technique relies on the identification of individual caspases without prior knowledge of their presence and activation in every cell type and species.

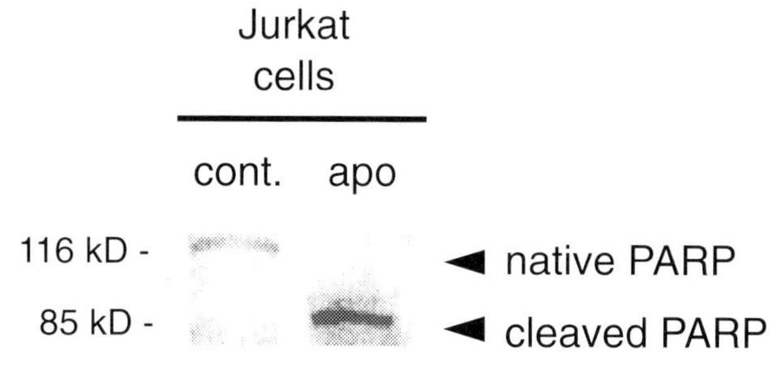

Figure 7.7
Cleavage of poly(ADP-ribose) polymerase (PARP) during apoptosis. Jurkat T lymphocytes were treated with phorbol 12-myristate 13-acetate and thapsigargin for 20 h to induce apoptosis. The cells were then subjected to SDS-polyacrylamide gel electrophoresis followed by immunoblotting with an antibody directed against PARP (band at ~114 kDa). PARP cleavage is shown by the appearance of a ~85 kDa band.

More common is the measurement of the cleavage of exogenously added or endogenous substrates. One of the most commonly assayed endogenous substrate assayed in apoptosis is the enzyme poly(ADP-ribose) polymerase (PARP) which is selectively cleaved by caspase-3 and related members to an approximately 85 kDa fragment, which can be detected by Western blot analysis (Figure 7.7; Lazebnik *et al.*, 1994). Although reported to occur in most cell types undergoing apoptosis, PARP cleavage to the 85 kDa fragment is also observed in some forms of necrosis (in addition to the formation of other PARP fragments) (Shah *et al.*, 1996) whereas PARP cleavage does not occur in hepatocytes dying by apoptosis (Jones *et al.*, 1998). Special precautions should be taken when studying apoptosis in mouse tissues since some secondary antibodies can cross-react with an 85 kDa protein that is unrelated to PARP (Budihardjo *et al.*, 1998). An alternative approach is to probe cytosolic extracts prepared from cells for caspase activity using specific tetrapeptides linked to a chromophore or fluorochrome such as benzyloxycarbonyl-Asp-Glu-Val-Asp-7-amino-4-trifluoromethylcoumarin (Z-DEVD-AFC). Upon cleavage of the tetrapeptide at the terminal Asp residue the chromophore or fluorochrome is liberated and becomes detectable by spectroscopy or fluorometry. The authors' laboratory has adapted this approach to the use of 96-well plates and a fluorescence plate reader, enabling the rapid screening of large numbers of samples.

While the assessment of apoptosis through biochemical assaying for caspase activation appears to be an attractive approach, we still know very little about the possible involvement of caspases in necrosis. Therefore, appropriate caution should be exercised when using caspase-based assays when screening the toxicity of novel drugs.

7.7 Choice of methods to study drug-induced apoptosis

As discussed earlier, drug-induced cytotoxicity may result in apoptosis, necrosis or a combination of both. Because of the generally reactive nature of a drug or its bioactivated proximate toxic form, multiple cellular components will often be targeted. The features of apoptosis may thus differ from the classical features observed following induction through a death receptor such as Fas. Consequently, any investigation of apoptosis, especially when dealing with drugs, should not rely on a single endpoint. Morphology remains the definite criterion for apoptosis and, although being time-consuming, should always be used to confirm any biochemical evidence for apoptosis.

Approaches based on annexin V and PI staining, detection of DNA fragmentation by the TUNEL assay or an immunoassay for nucleosomes are extremely powerful and have the potential to be adapted to rapid screening programmes. Some also have a relatively good discrimination power between apoptosis and necrosis. However, a major problem remains the degeneration of apoptotic cells into secondary necrotic cells, which is often difficult to distinguish biochemically from primary necrosis. In many lymphoid cells, chromatin condensation and apoptotic body formation following treatment with glucocorticoids or activation of death receptors are very clearly defined and can be made detectable by modern image analysis equipment. In the case of cells from solid tissues or growing in monolayers, the nuclear changes may be less pronounced. For instance, apoptotic body formation is a late event in hepatocytes undergoing apoptosis through Fas stimulation, where instead the nuclei initially become highly shrunken (pyknotic) (Jones *et al.*, 1998). Another complication is that adherent cells, when undergoing apoptosis, have the tendency to detach from the substratum on which they grow. While cultured neurones and hepatocytes remain adherent during the early phases of apoptosis, endothelial cells display nuclear chromatin condensation only after they have detached from the dish on which they are cultured (Bonfoco *et al.*, 1997; Kass and Jones, unpublished observations).

7.8 Conclusions

Our understanding of the causes and mechanisms of cytotoxicity has advanced greatly during the past decade. The number of experimental approaches to study cell death has increased proportionally, and, with the rapidly increasing interest in apoptosis research, numerous commercial companies are now offering kits for the rapid screening for cell death. Despite these advances, the differentiation between apoptosis and necrosis remains a challenge. Future research efforts should therefore focus to identify endpoints that are unambiguous and distinguish between apoptosis and necrosis (primary and secondary to apoptosis), and that can be easily incorporated into throughput screening programmes.

Future research efforts should focus to identify endpoints that are unambiguous and distinguish between apoptosis and necrosis, and that can be easily incorporated into throughput screening programmes.

Acknowledgements

We are grateful to Dr J. Fred Nagelkerke (Leiden University, The Netherlands) for kindly providing us with flow cytometric annexin V binding data (Figure 7.5) and Dr Diana Toivola (Stanford University, USA) for critical comments. The work from the authors' laboratory cited here was supported in part by the Swedish Medical Research Council and MRC (UK).

References

Afanasyev, V.N., Korol, B.A., Matylevich, N.P., Pechatnikov, V.A. and Umansky, S.R., 1993, The use of flow cytometry for the investigation of cell death, *Cytometry*, **14**, 603–609.

Andree, H.A.M., Reutelingsperger, C.P.M., Hauptmann, R., Hemker, H.C., Hermens, W.T. and Willems, G.M., 1990, Binding of vascular anticoagulant-alpha (vac-α) to planar phospholipid-bilayers, *Journal of Biological Chemistry*, **265**, 4923–4928.

Ankarcrona, M., Dypbukt, J.M., Bonfoco, E., Zhivotovsky, B., Orrenius, S., Lipton, S.A. *et al.*, 1995, Glutamate-induced neuronal death: a succession of necrosis or apoptosis depending on mitochondrial function, *Neuron*, **15**, 961–973.

Arends, M.J. and Wyllie, A.H., 1991, Apoptosis: mechanisms and roles in pathology, *International Review of Experimental Pathology*, **32**, 223–254.

Bicknell, G.R. and Cohen, G.M., 1995, Cleavage of DNA to large kilobase pair fragments occurs in some forms of necrosis as well as apoptosis, *Biochemical and Biophysical Research Communications*, **207**, 40–47.

Blazka, M.E., Elwell, M.R., Holladay, S.D., Wilson, R.E. and Luster, M.I., 1996, Histopathology of acetaminophen-induced liver changes: role of interleukin-1α and tumor necrosis factor α, *Toxicologic Pathology*, **24**, 181–189.

Bonfoco, E., Krainc, D., Ankarcrona, M., Nicotera, P. and Lipton, S.A., 1995, Apoptosis and necrosis: two distinct events induced, respectively, by mild and intense insults with *N*-methyl-D-aspartate or nitric oxide/superoxide in cortical cell cultures, *Proceedings of the National Academy of Sciences U.S.A.*, **92**, 7162–7166.

Bonfoco, E., Ankarcrona, M., Krainc, D., Nicotera, P. and Lipton, S.A., 1997, Techniques for distinguishing apoptosis from necrosis in cerebrocortical and cerebellar neurons. In: *Apoptosis Techniques and Protocols*, 237–253. Edited by Poirier, J. Totowa, New Jersey, Humana Press.

Brown, D.G., Sun, X.-M. and Cohen, G.M., 1993, Dexamethasone-induced apoptosis involves cleavage of DNA to large fragments prior to internucleosomal fragmentation, *Journal of Biological Chemistry*, **268**, 3037–3039.

Bruno, S., Lassota, P., Giaretti, W. and Darzynkiewicz, Z., 1992, Apoptosis of rat thymocytes triggered by prednisolone, camptothecin, or teniposide is selective to G_0 cells and is prevented by inhibitors of proteases, *Oncology Research*, **4**, 29–35.

Budihardjo, I.I., Poirier, G.G. and Kaufmann, S.H., 1998, Apparent cleavage of poly(ADP-ribose) polymerase in nonapoptotic mouse lta cells: an artifact of cross-reactive secondary antibody, *Molecular and Cellular Biochemistry*, **178**, 245–249.

Cohen, G.M., Sun, X.-M., Snowden, R.T., Dinsdale, D. and Skilleter, D.N., 1992, Key morphological features of apoptosis may occur in the absence of internucleosomal DNA fragmentation, *The Biochemical Journal*, **286**, 331–334.

Cohen, G.M., 1997, Caspases: the executioners of apoptosis, *The Biochemical Journal*, **326**, 1–16.

Cohen, J.J. and Duke, R.C., 1984, Glucocorticoid activation of a calcium-dependent endonuclease in thymocyte nuclei leads to cell death, *Journal of Immunology*, **132**, 38–42.

Darzynkiewicz, Z., Juan, G., Li, X., Gorczyca, W., Murakami, T. and Traganos, F., 1997, Cytometry in cell necrobiology: analysis of apoptosis and accidental cell death (necrosis), *Cytometry*, **27**, 1–20.

Decaudin, D., Geley, S., Hirsch, T., Castedo, M., Marchetti, P., Macho, A. *et al.*, 1997, Bcl-2 and bcl-x(l) antagonize the mitochondrial dysfunction preceding nuclear apoptosis induced by chemotherapeutic agents, *Cancer Research*, **57**, 62–67.

Dong, Z., Saikumar, P., Weinberg, J.M. and Venkatachalam, M.A., 1997, Internucleosomal DNA cleavage triggered by plasma membrane damage during necrotic cell death: involvement of serine but not cysteine proteases, *American Journal of Pathology*, **151**, 1205–1213.

Dypbukt, J.M., Ankarcrona, M., Burkitt, M., Sjöholm, Å., Ström, K., Orrenius, S. *et al.*, 1994, Different prooxidant levels stimulate growth, trigger apoptosis, or produce necrosis of insulin-secreting RINm5F cells: the role of intracellular polyamines, *Journal of Biological Chemistry*, **269**, 30553–30560.

Ellis, R.E., Yuan, J. and Horvitz, H.R., 1991, Mechanisms and functions of cell death, *Annual Review of Cell Biology*, **7**, 663–698.

Enari, M., Sakahira, H., Yokoyama, H., Okawa, K., Iwamatsu, A. and Nagata, S., 1998, A caspase-activated DNase that degrades DNA during apoptosis, and its inhibitor ICAD, *Nature*, **391**, 43–50.

Ernst, M., 1926, Über Untergang von Zellen während der normalen Entwicklung bei Wirbeltieren, *Zeitschrift für Anatomische Entwicklungsgeschichte*, **79**, 228–262.

Fadok, V.A., Voelker, D.R., Campbell, P.A., Cohen, J.J., Bratton, D.L. and Henson, P.M., 1992, Exposure of phosphatidylserine on the surface of apoptotic lymphocytes triggers specific recognition and removal by macrophages, *Journal of Immunology*, **148**, 2207–2216.

Fesus, L., Thomazy, V. and Falus, A., 1987, Induction and activation of tissue transglutaminase during programmed cell death, *FEBS Letters*, **224**, 104–108.

Filipski, J., Leblanc, J., Youdale, T., Sikorska, M. and Walker, P.R., 1990, Periodicity of DNA folding in higher order chromatin structures, *EMBO Journal*, **9**, 1319–1327.

Fischer-Nielsen, A., Corcoran, G.B., Poulsen, H.E., Kamendulis, L.M. and Loft, S., 1995, Menadione-induced DNA fragmentation without 8-oxo-2′-deoxyguanosine formation in isolated rat hepatocytes, *Biochemical Pharmacology*, **49**, 1469–1474.

Froelich, C.J., Dixit, V.M. and Yang, X.H., 1998, Lymphocyte granule-mediated apoptosis: matters of viral mimicry and deadly proteases, *Immunology Today*, **19**, 30–36.

Galle, P.R., Hofmann, W.J., Walczak, H., Schaller, H., Otto, G., Stremmel, W. *et al.*, 1995, Involvement of the CD95 (APO-1/Fas) receptor and ligand in liver-damage, *Journal of Experimental Medicine*, **182**, 1223–1230.

Gavrieli, Y., Sherman, Y. and Bensasson, S.A., 1992, Identification of programmed cell death in situ via specific labeling of nuclear DNA fragmentation, *Journal of Cell Biology*, **119**, 493–501.

Glücksmann, A., 1951, Cell death in normal vertebrate ontogeny, *Biological Reviews*, **26**, 59–86.

Goldin, R.D., Ratnayaka, I.D., Breach, C.S., Brown, I.N. and Wickramasinghe, S.N., 1996, Role of macrophages in acetaminophen (paracetamol)-induced hepatotoxicity, *Journal of Pathology*, **179**, 432–435.

Gorczyca, W., Bruno, S., Darzynkiewicz, R.J., Gong, J.P. and Darzynkiewicz, Z., 1992, DNA strand breaks occurring during apoptosis: their early in situ detection by the terminal deoxynucleotidyl transferase and nick translation assays and prevention by serine protease inhibitors, *International Journal of Oncology*, **1**, 639–648.

Gorczyca, W., Bigman, K., Mittelman, A., Ahmed, T., Gong, J.P., Melamed, M.R. *et al.*, 1993, Induction of DNA strand breaks associated with apoptosis during treatment of leukemias, *Leukemia*, **7**, 659–670.

Hannun, Y.A., 1996, Functions of ceramide in coordinating cellular responses to stress, *Science*, **274**, 1855–1859.

Herr, I., Wilhelm, D., Bohler, T., Angel, P. and Debatin, K.-M., 1997, Activation of CD95 (APO-1/Fas) signaling by ceramide mediates cancer therapy-induced apoptosis, *EMBO Journal*, **16**, 6200–6208.

Jacobson, M.D., Weil, M. and Raff, M.C., 1997, Programmed cell death in animal development, *Cell*, **88**, 347–354.

Jewell, S.A., Bellomo, G., Thorn, P., Orrenius, S. and Smith, M.T., 1982, Bleb formation in hepatocytes during drug metabolism is caused by disturbances in thiol and calcium ion homeostasis, *Science*, **217**, 1257–1259.

Jones, R.A., Johnson, V.L., Buck, N.R., Dobrota, M., Hinton, R.H., Chow, S.C. *et al.*, 1998, Fas-mediated apoptosis in mouse hepatocytes involves the processing and activation of caspases, *Hepatology*, **27**, 1632–1642.

Kane, D.J., Sarafian, T.A., Anton, R., Hahn, H., Gralla, E.B., Valentine, J.S. *et al.*, 1993, Bcl-2 inhibition of neural death: decreased generation of reactive oxygen species, *Science*, **262**, 1274–1277.

Kane, D.J., Ord, T., Anton, R. and Bredesen, D.E., 1995, Expression of bcl-2 inhibits necrotic neural cell-death, *Journal of Neuroscience Research*, **40**, 269–275.

Kass, G.E.N., Wright, J.M., Nicotera, P. and Orrenius, S., 1988, The mechanism of 1-methyl-4-phenyl-1,2,3,6-tetrahydropyridine toxicity: role of intracellular calcium, *Archives of Biochemistry and Biophysics*, **260**, 789–797.

Kass, G.E.N., Juedes, M.J. and Orrenius, S., 1992, Cyclosporin A protects hepatocytes against prooxidant-induced cell killing. A study on the role of mitochondrial Ca^{2+} cycling in cytotoxicity, *Biochemical Pharmacology*, **44**, 1995–2003.

Kass, G.E.N., Eriksson, J.E., Weis, M., Orrenius, S. and Chow, S.C., 1996, Chromatin condensation during apoptosis requires ATP, *The Biochemical Journal*, **318**, 749–752.

Kass, G.E.N. and Orrenius, S., 1999, Calcium signaling and cytotoxicity, *Environmental Health Perspectives*, **107**, 25–35.

Kaufmann, S.H., 1989, Induction of endonucleolytic DNA cleavage in human acute myelogenous leukemia-cells by etoposide, camptothecin, and other cytotoxic anticancer drugs – a cautionary note, *Cancer Research*, **49**, 5870–5878.

Kerr, J.F.R., Wyllie, A.H. and Currie, A.R., 1972, Apoptosis: a basic biological phenomenon with wide-ranging implications in tissue kinetics, *British Journal of Cancer*, **26**, 239–257.

Kerr, J.F.R., Searle, J., Harmon, B.V. and Bishop, C.J., 1987, Apoptosis, in: *Perspectives on Mammalian Cell Death*, 93–128, edited by Potten, C.S., Oxford: Oxford University Press.

Kondo, T., Suda, T., Fukuyama, H., Adachi, M. and Nagata, S., 1997, Essential roles of the Fas ligand in the development of hepatitis, *Nature Medicine*, **3**, 409–413.

Koopman, G., Reutelingsperger, C.P.M., Kuijten, G.A.M., Keehnen, R.M.J., Pals, S.T. and Vanoers, M.H.J., 1994, Annexin-V for flow cytometric detection of phosphatidylserine expression on B-cells undergoing apoptosis, *Blood*, **84**, 1415–1420.

Kroemer, G., Zamzami, N. and Susin, S.A., 1997, Mitochondrial control of apoptosis, *Immunology Today*, **18**, 44–51.

Laskin, D.L., 1996, Sinusoidal lining cells and hepatotoxicity, *Toxicologic Pathology*, **24**, 112–118.

Lazebnik, Y.A., Kaufmann, S.H., Desnoyers, S., Poirier, G.G. and Earnshaw, W.C., 1994, Cleavage of poly(ADP-ribose) polymerase by a proteinase with properties like ICE, *Nature*, **371**, 346–347.

Leist, M., Gantner, F., Bohlinger, I., Tiegs, G. and Wendel, A., 1994, Application of the cell death ELISA for the detection of tumor necrosis factor-induced DNA fragmentation in murine models of inflammatory organ failure, *Biochemica*, **3**, 18–20.

Leist, M., Single, B., Castoldi, A.F., Kuhnle, S. and Nicotera, P., 1997, Intracellular adenosine triphosphate (ATP) concentration: a switch in the decision between apoptosis and necrosis, *Journal of Experimental Medicine*, **185**, 1481–1486.

Li, X., Traganos, F., Melamed, M.R. and Darzynkiewicz, Z., 1995, Single-step procedure for labeling DNA strand breaks with fluorescein-conjugated or BODIPY-conjugated deoxynucleotides: detection of apoptosis and bromodeoxyuridine incorporation, *Cytometry*, **20**, 172–180.

Liu, X., Li, P., Widlak, P., Zou, H., Luo, X., Garrard, W.T. and Wang, X., 1998, The 40-kDa subunit of DNA fragmentation factor induces DNA fragmentation and chromatin condensation during apoptosis, *Journal of Biological Chemistry*, **95**, 8461–8466.

Lockshin, R.A. and Williams, C.M., 1965, Programmed cell death. I. Cytology of degeneration in the intersegmented muscles of the Pernyi silkmoth, *Journal of Insect Physiology*, **11**, 123–133.

Majno, G. and Joris, I., 1995, Apoptosis, oncosis, and necrosis – an overview of cell-death, *American Journal of Pathology*, **146**, 3–15.

Meyn, R.E., Stephens, L.C., Hunter, N.R. and Milas, L., 1994, Induction of apoptosis in murine tumors by cyclophosphamide, *Cancer Chemotherapy and Pharmacology*, **33**, 410–414.

Meyn, R.E., Stephens, L.C., Hunter, N.R. and Milas, L., 1995, Apoptosis in murine tumors treated with chemotherapy agents, *Anti-Cancer Drugs*, **6**, 443–450.

Moreira, L.F., Naomoto, Y., Hamada, M., Kamikawa, Y. and Orita, K., 1995, Assessment of apoptosis in esophageal-carcinoma preoperatively treated by chemotherapy and radiotherapy, *Anticancer Research*, **15**, 639–644.

Murgia, M., Pizzo, P., Sandona, D., Zanovello, P., Rizzuto, R. and Di Virgilio, F., 1992, Mitochondrial DNA is not fragmented during apoptosis, *Journal of Biological Chemistry*, **267**, 10939–10941.

Nagata, S., 1997, Apoptosis by death factor, *Cell*, **88**, 355–365.

Nicholson, D.W. and Thornberry, N.A., 1997, Caspases: killer proteases, *Trends in Biochemical Sciences*, **22**, 299–306.

Oberhammer, F., Wilson, J.W., Dive, C., Morris, I.D., Hickman, J.A., Wakeling, A.E. *et al.*, 1993, Apoptotic death in epithelial cells: cleavage of DNA to 300 and/or 50 kb fragments prior to or in the absence of internucleosomal fragmentation, *EMBO Journal*, **12**, 3679–3684.

Ogasawara, J., Watanabe Fukunaga, R., Adachi, M., Matsuzawa, A., Kasugai, T., Kitamura, Y. *et al.*, 1993, Lethal effect of the anti-Fas antibody in mice, *Nature*, **364**, 806–809.

Ormerod, M.G., Collins, M.K.L., Rodriguez-Tarduchy, G. and Robertson, D., 1992, Apoptosis in interleukin-3-dependent hematopoietic cells: quantification by two flow cytometric methods, *Journal of Immunological Methods*, **153**, 57–65.

Ormerod, M.G., Sun, X.M., Snowden, R.T., Davies, R., Fearnhead, H. and Cohen, G.M., 1993, Increased membrane-permeability of apoptotic thymocytes – a flow cytometric study, *Cytometry*, **14**, 595–602.

Ormerod, M.G., O'Neill, C.F., Robertson, D. and Harrap, K.R., 1994a, Cisplatin induces apoptosis in a human ovarian-carcinoma cell-line without concomitant internucleosomal degradation of DNA, *Experimental Cell Research*, **211**, 231–237.

Ormerod, M.G., Orr, R.M. and Peacock, J.H., 1994b, The role of apoptosis in cell-killing by cisplatin – a flow cytometric study, *British Journal of Cancer*, **69**, 93–100.

Patel, T., Arora, A. and Gores, G.J., 1995, A fluorometric assay for quantitating DNA strand breaks during apoptosis, *Analytical Biochemistry*, **229**, 229–235.

Raffray, M. and Cohen, G.M., 1997, Apoptosis and necrosis in toxicology: a continuum or distinct modes of cell death?, *Pharmacology and Therapeutics*, **75**, 153–177.

Ray, S.D., Kamendulis, L.M., Gurule, M.W., Yorkin, R.D. and Corcoran, G.B., 1993, Ca^{2+} antagonists inhibit DNA fragmentation and toxic cell death induced by acetaminophen, *FASEB Journal*, **7**, 453–463.

Rosser, B.G. and Gores, G.J., 1995, Liver cell necrosis: cellular mechanisms and clinical implications, *Gastroenterology*, **108**, 252–275.

Rudin, C.M. and Thompson, C.B., 1997, Apoptosis and disease: regulation and clinical relevance of programmed cell death, *Annual Review of Medicine*, **48**, 267–281.

Saunders, J.W., 1966, Death in the embryonic system, *Science*, **154**, 604–612.

Schwartz, L.M., Smith, S.W., Jones, M.E.E. and Osborne, B.A., 1993, Do all programmed cell deaths occur via apoptosis, *Proceedings of the National Academy of Sciences U.S.A.*, **90**, 980–984.

Shah, G.M., Shah, R.G. and Poirier, G.G., 1996, Different cleavage pattern for poly(ADP-ribose) polymerase during necrosis and apoptosis in HL-60 cells, *Biochemical and Biophysical Research Communications*, **229**, 838–844.

Shimizu, S., Eguchi, Y., Kamiike, W., Waguri, S., Uchiyama, Y., Matsuda, H. *et al.* and Tsujimoto, Y., 1996, Retardation of chemical hypoxia-induced necrotic cell-death by bcl-2 and ICE inhibitors – possible involvement of common mediators in apoptotic and necrotic signal transductions, *Oncogene*, **12**, 2045–2050.

Sorenson, C.M., Barry, M.A. and Eastman, A., 1990, Analysis of events associated with cell cycle arrest at G2 phase and cell death induced by cisplatin, *Journal of the National Cancer Institute*, **82**, 749–755.

Strasser, A., Harris, A.W. and Cory, S., 1991, Bcl-2 transgene inhibits T cell death and perturbs thymic self-censorship, *Cell*, **67**, 889–899.

Su, I.J., Cheng, A.L., Tsai, T.F. and Lay, J.D., 1993, Retinoic acid-induced apoptosis and regression of a refractory Epstein-Barr virus-containing T-cell lymphoma expressing multidrug-resistance phenotypes, *British Journal of Haematology*, **85**, 826–828.

Sun, X.-M. and Cohen, G.M. 1994, Mg^{2+}-dependent cleavage of DNA into kilobase pair fragments is responsible for the initial degradation of DNA in apoptosis, *Journal of Biological Chemistry*, **269**, 14857–14860.

Telford, W.G., King, L.E. and Fraker, P.J., 1994, Rapid quantitation of apoptosis in pure and heterogeneous cell populations using flow-cytometry, *Journal of Immunological Methods*, **172**, 1–16.

Thompson, C.B., 1995, Apoptosis in the pathogenesis and treatment of disease, *Science*, **267**, 1456–1462.

Tomei, L.D., Kanter, P. and Wenner, C.E., 1988, Inhibition of radiation-induced apoptosis in vitro by tumor promoters, *Biochemical and Biophysical Research Communications*, **155**, 324–331.

Trump, B.F., Berezesky, I.K., Chang, S.H. and Phelps, P.C., 1997, The pathways of cell death: oncosis, apoptosis, and necrosis, *Toxicologic Pathology*, **25**, 82–88.

Villa, P., Kaufmann, S.H. and Earnshaw, W.C., 1997, Caspases and caspase inhibitors, *Trends in Biochemical Sciences*, **22**, 388–393.

Walker, P.R., Smith, C., Youdale, T., Leblanc, J., Whitfield, J.F. and Sikorska, M., 1991, Topoisomerase-II-reactive chemotherapeutic drugs induce apoptosis in thymocytes, *Cancer Research*, **51**, 1078–1085.

Weis, M., Kass, G.E.N. and Orrenius, S., 1994, Further characterization of the events involved in mitochondrial Ca^{2+} release and pore formation by prooxidants, *Biochemical Pharmacology*, **47**, 2147–2156.

Weis, M., Schlegel, J., Kass, G.E.N., Holmström, T.H., Peters, I., Eriksson, J. *et al.*, 1995, Cellular events in Fas/APO-1-mediated apoptosis in JURKAT T lymphocytes, *Experimental Cell Research*, **219**, 699–708.

Wyllie, A.H., 1980, Glucocorticoid-induced thymocyte apoptosis is associated with endogenous endonuclease activation, *Nature*, **284**, 555–556.

Zhivotovsky, B., Nicotera, P., Bellomo, G., Hanson, K. and Orrenius, S., 1993, Ca^{2+} and endonuclease activation in radiation-induced lymphoid cell death, *Experimental Cell Research*, **207**, 163–170.

Zhivotovsky, B., Cedervall, B., Jiang, S., Nicotera, P. and Orrenius, S., 1994, Involvement of Ca^{2+} in the formation of high molecular weight DNA fragments in thymocyte apoptosis, *Biochemical and Biophysical Research Communications*, **202**, 120–127.

8 Genetically Modified Cells to Assess Drug Metabolism *In Vitro*

Mikael Oscarson and Magnus Ingelman-Sundberg, Institute of Environmental Medicine, Stockholm, Sweden

8.1 Introduction

8.1.1 Principles in drug metabolism

Most pharmacologically active compounds are lipophilic and will be reabsorbed in the kidneys after glomerular filtration. Excretion of these compounds is facilitated by biotransformation in phase 1 and phase 2 reactions that convert them into more polar substances. In the phase 1 reactions, functional groups are introduced or modified by either dehydrogenation, oxidation, reduction, hydrolysis or hydroxylation. The phase 1 enzymes include cytochromes P450, mono-aminoxidase, microsomal flavine-containing monooxygenase, alcohol- and aldehyde dehydrogenases, aldehyde oxidases, esterases and epoxid hydrolases. In the phase 2 reactions carried out by the UDP-glucuronolsyltransferases (UGTs), glutathione S transferases (GSTs), sulphotransferases and N-acetyltransferases (NATs), the functional groups are modified in glucuronidation, glutathione, sulphation, or acetylation conjugation reactions that usually result in the formation of more polar compounds that are more readily excreted from the body. Many of these drug metabolizing enzymes (DMEs) are localized in the membranes of the endoplasmic reticulum, although the dehydrogenases, sulphotransferases and acetyltransferases are cytosolic. Accumulating evidence reveals that the liver is by far the most quantitatively important organ for these reactions.

In order to meet the structural diversity of the substrate chemicals, all these enzymes exist in multiple forms with different but often partially overlapping substrate specificities and generally 5–30 different genes encoding drug metabolizing enzymes are present.

8.1.2 Preclinical studies of drug metabolism

Today it has become evident that it is beneficial to devote much effort early in the drug development process, long before exposure to humans, to characterize the pharmacokinetic aspect of the NCE (new chemical entity). Important aspects of early prediction of human drug metabolism includes absorption, bioavailability and clearance. Many of the candidate drugs are withdrawn only because of too high clearance, and subtle modifications of the chemical structure can often change the rate of metabolism without affecting the pharmacological properties.

The main initial topics to be dealt with early in development are the solubility of the compound, the rate of absorption and the metabolic stability. In the preclinical phases, early identification of the active or reactive metabolites is advantageous as well as identification of the metabolic pathways of the compound. Furthermore, inter-species comparisons of the drug metabolism should be carried out, the enzymes responsible for the metabolism should be assigned, the occurrence of polymorphic enzymes in its important pathways of biotransformation should be evaluated, the possibility that the compound is an inhibitor or an inducer of the enzymes should be explored and the kind of drug–drug interactions identified.

Of all NCEs being evaluated in the drug discovery process, up to 33% are withdrawn because of unwanted pharmacokinetic properties, and an additional 20% are withdrawn because of toxicity in laboratory animals or in humans (Monro, 1996). An early prediction of drug metabolism and pharmacokinetic parameters as well as toxicity would therefore be useful in that it can assist in the selection of appropriate candidate drugs and thereby shorten the development process and reduce the costs. In addition, knowledge of drug metabolism is essential for prediction of interindividual differences in metabolism and of drug–drug interactions, a fact which has also been acknowledged by the regulatory agencies (FDA, 1997).

Knowledge about the enzyme specificity of a drug thus has important implications for the prediction of drug–drug interactions at the level of metabolism (Li, 1997). This can be exemplified with the terfenadine–ketoconazole interaction, where patients receiving concurrent treatment with the H$_1$-histamine antagonist terfenadine and the antifungal agent ketoconazole developed life-threatening cardiac arrhythmias (*torsades de pointes*). The molecular explanation is that ketoconazole is a potent inhibitor of CYP3A4, the major catalyst of terfenadine, thus causing higher plasma concentrations of the parent drug and predisposing for the ventricular arrhythmias (Woosley *et al.*, 1993). Using *in vitro* methods this interaction could have been predicted (von Moltke *et al.*, 1994b), and with the knowledge of enzyme specificity, interaction between these drugs and other CYP3A4 substrates can be anticipated.

The appreciation of all the important aspects regarding drug metabolism and drug–drug interactions requires that the specific enzyme responsible for that metabolism is identified. For this purpose, different *in vitro* systems can be used. The biological systems include subcellular systems, primary cells in culture, transformed cell lines, tissue slices and recombinant expressed enzymes. With respect to interactions with specific forms of P450 or other drug metabolizing enzymes, it is evident that the recombinantly expressed cDNA-systems represents the most informative system.

In this chapter we describe the characteristics and usefulness of the various heterologous systems for expression of drug metabolizing enzymes with emphasis on their use in drug development.

8.1.3 *The major human cyctochromes P450 in drug metabolism – general characteristics*

It is becoming increasingly evident that only a limited number of different cytochrome P450-forms account for the majority of P450-dependent phase 1 metabolism of clinically used drugs: CYP1A2, CYP2A6, CYP2C9, CYP2C19, CYP2D6, CYP2E1 and CYP3A4 (see Figure 8.1). Based on the evaluation of clearance of 315 drugs, Bertz and Granneman (1997) concluded that 56% of those were primarily cleared by P450 and, of those, over 85% were metabolized by either CYP2C9/19, CYP2D6 or CYP3A4. In 26% of the cases of P450-dependent metabolism the specific P450 form responsible for the metabolism could not be identified. The enzyme specificity for clinically used drugs has also been reviewed by Rendic and Di Carlo (1997).

The drug metabolizing forms of P450s are localized on five different chromosomes and their marker substrates for *in vivo* evaluation are given in Table 8.2. It is evident that the majority of these enzymes are both polymorphic and inducible (cf. Table 8.1), thereby contributing to the important

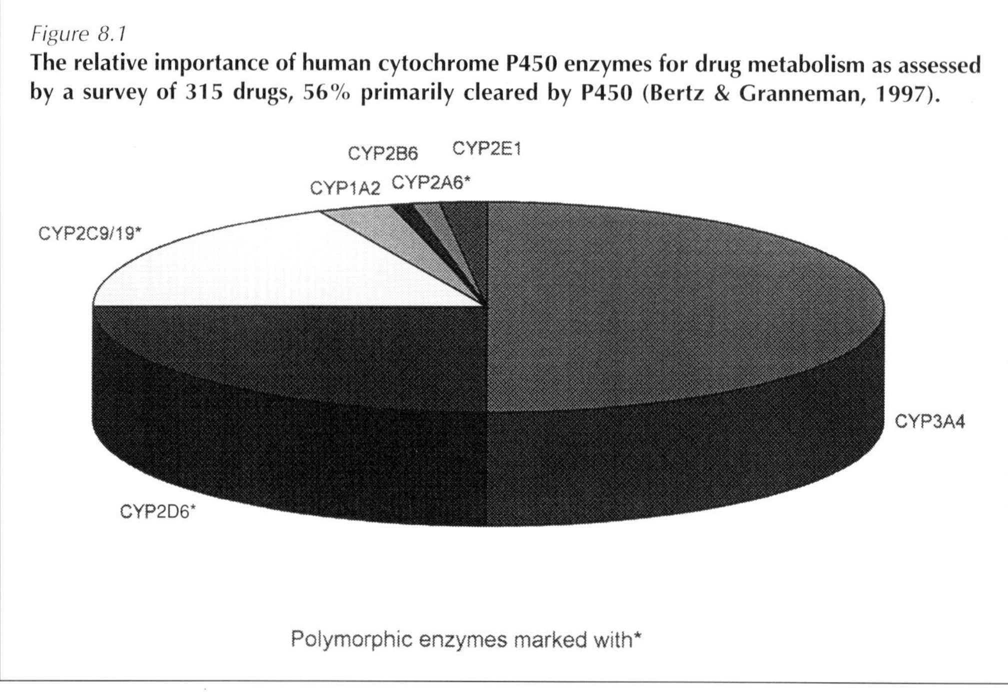

Figure 8.1

The relative importance of human cytochrome P450 enzymes for drug metabolism as assessed by a survey of 315 drugs, 56% primarily cleared by P450 (Bertz & Granneman, 1997).

Table 8.1   Major human P450s participating in drug metabolism

Enzyme	Chromosomal localization	Polymorphic	Inducible
CYP1A2	15q22	No	Yes
CYP2A6	19q13	Yes	Yes
CYP2C9	10q24	Yes	Yes
CYP2C19	10q24	Yes	Yes
CYP2D6	22q13	Yes	No
CYP2E1	10q24	(Yes)	Yes
CYP3A4	7q22	No	Yes

interindividual differences in enzyme expression and rate of drug metabolism.

The contribution of various P450 forms to the metabolism of a particular drug can be examined *in vitro* using different inhibitors and its activity *in vivo* can be monitored using relatively specific probe drugs for the various enzymes as outlined in Table 8.2.

The P450-dependent hydroxylation reaction requires two electrons donated from NADPH via the flavoprotein NADPH-cytochrome P450 reductase and in some cases also cytochrome b_5. In the process, dioxygen is reduced to water and the substrate oxidized. In the human liver microsomal

Table 8.2   Human drug metabolizing P450s – marker activities and inhibitors for *in vitro* use

Enzyme	Marker activity	Inhibitor
CYP1A2	Ethoxyresorufin-*O*-deethylation	Fluvoxamine
	Phenacetin-*O*-deethylation	Furafylline
CYP2A6	Coumarin-7-hydroxylation	
CYP2C9	Diclofenac-4′-hydroxylation	Sulfaphenazole
	S-Warfarin-7-hydroxylation	
CYP2C19	*S*-Mephenytoin-4′-hydroxylation	
	R-Omeprazole-5-hydroxylation	
CYP2D6	Debrisoquine-4-hydroxylation	Quinidine
	Bufuralol-1′-hydroxylation	
	Dextromethorphan-*N*-demethylation	
CYP2E1	Chlorzoxazone-6-hydroxylation	4-Methylpyrazole
		Diehyldithiocarbamate
CYP3A4	Testosterone-6β-hydroxylation	Ketoconazole
	Nifedipine oxidation	

membrane, the total molar quantity of P450 is about 10–20 fold higher than that of the reductase, whereas in many cDNA expressed systems this ratio approaches 1. Different forms of P450 vary in their preference for cytochrome b_5. In some cases the action of b_5 is stimulatory, in some cases inhibitory, an outcome that also depends on the particular substrate. The action of cytochrome b_5 could also be only allosteric in nature. The multiple roles of b_5 must thus be taken to account and treated individually in the different cDNA expression systems.

There are important interspecies differences in the properties, regulation and substrate specificities of the hepatic drug metabolizing P450s. This fact complicates extrapolation of results regarding metabolic pathways and rate of metabolism as well as the formation of potentially toxic or pharmacologically active metabolites, e.g. from rodent and dog models to humans.

The major characteristics of the drug metabolizing human P450s are as follows (see Ingelman-Sundberg, 1997b; Ingelman-Sundberg and Johansson, 1995; Parkinson, 1996; Wrighton *et al.*, 1996, for a detailed description).

8.1.3.1   *CYP1A2*

CYP1A2 is involved in the metabolism of acetaminophen, aromatic amines, caffeine, phenacetin and theophylline. However several of these drugs are also substrate for other enzymes. To a great extent the substrate specificity of CYP1A2 with respect to the metabolism of more hydrophilic compounds resembles that of CYP2E1. Specific inhibitors of CYP1A2 are, for example, furafylline and fluvoxamine. The enzyme is induced by smoking, Brussels sprouts and charbroiled beef.

8.1.3.2 *CYP2A6*

CYP2A6, originally identified as coumarin hydroxylase, participates in the metabolism of only a few drugs, among them fadrozole, letrozole, methoxyflurane and losigamone. It metabolizes nicotine and some carcinogenic compounds like aflatoxin B1 and NNK. There are two defective alleles (v1 and v2) present at allele frequences between 2–30% in different populations (Fernandez-Salguero *et al.*, 1995).

8.1.3.3 *CYP2C9*

CYP2C9 accepts both acids and bases of substrates, and among the important substrates are acetylsalicylic acid, diclophenac, indomethacin, naproxen, fenytoin, tolbutamide and warfarin. The amino acid sequence is very similar to that of CYP2C19, although their substrate specificities differ. CYP2C9 is highly inducible by rifampicin. Two different allelic variants of the *CYP2C9* gene had been described. One causing R144C leads to impaired interactions with P450 reductase and one resulting in I359L causes less productive interactions with some of the substrates. The latter mutation appears to be more clinically relevant, in particular because of the narrow therapeutic range of some of the CYP2C9 substrates like warfarin.

8.1.3.4 *CYP2C19*

The importance of CYP2C19 is growing in terms of the number of drug substrates and approximately 15 different specific CYP2C19 drug substrates are known at the present time, e.g. citalopram, diazepam, hexobarbital, imipramine, proguanil and propranolol. CYP2C19 is also inducible by rifampicin and possible by barbiturates, causing large inter-individual variability in AUC for these drugs. Four different defective alleles of *CYP2C19* have been described but two (*CYP2C19*2* and *CYP2C19*3*) account for the majority of the poor metabolizer phenotype within most populations.

8.1.3.5 *CYP2D6*

CYP2D6 might be responsible for about 30% of the drug metabolism of clinically used drugs known today. The enzyme metabolizes antidepressants, neuroleptics, β-blockers as well as codeine, dextrometorphan, ethylmorphine and nicotine. Bases with a planar hydrophobic part are relatively specific substrates for this enzyme. Drug–drug interactions are clinically relevant, for example between serotonin reuptake inhibitors and tricyclic antidepressants. The enzyme appears to be induced during pregnancy (Wadelius *et al.*, 1997). About 7% of the Caucasian population lacks functional enzyme, whereas 2–30% of different populations in the world are ultrarapid metabolizers of CYP2D6 and have multiple gene copies (Ingelman-Sundberg, 1997a).

8.1.3.6   CYP2E1

CYP2E1 has an important endogenous role in the metabolism of acetone to gluconeogenetic precursors and provides the only drug metabolizing P450 where a major physiological function is known. CYP2E1 is mainly of toxicological importance and participates in the metabolic activation of nitrosoamines, organic solvents, some drugs and of alcohol. The cellular level of CYP2E1 is increased in the presence of its substrates, mainly because of post-translational stabilization. Among the most potent inducers in humans are ethanol and isoniazid. The enzyme is not functionally polymorphic to a great extent and we have only found one functionally different allele which is very rare (Hu *et al.*, 1997). There are some inhibitors of CYP2E1, e.g. diethyldithiocarbonate, dibromoethane, disulfiram, ethanol and chlormethiazole (cf. Ronis *et al.*, 1996). The latter compound appears to be an effective inhibitor also *in vivo* in man (Gebhardt *et al.*, 1997). The enzyme metabolizes many different compounds, e.g. acetaminophen, caffeine, chloroform, chlorzoxazone, dapsone, enflurane, halothane, which usually are small and hydrophobic in nature.

8.1.3.7   CYP3A4

CYP3A4 is the most important P450 enzyme in the metabolism of drugs, with more then 60 known different substrates. The substrate binding pocket accepts very large compounds. There are quite potent inhibitors of CYP3A4 such as chlotrimazole, ketoconazole and troleandomycin. Furthermore, the enzyme is highly inducible by, for example, barbiturates, dexamethasone, fenytoin and rifampicin. No genetic polymorphism of CYP3A4 has been described and the protein is to a great extent regulated in a similar manner as P-glycoprotein. The genes are also localized on the same

Table 8.3   The polymorphic human xenobiotic metabolizing P450 enzymes

Enzyme	Major detrimental mutation	Consequence	Frequency of the major mutant allele in Caucasians (%)
CYP2A6	Leu160→His	Defect enzyme	5%
CYP2C9	Arg144→Cys	Enzyme with impaired interactions with reductase	20%
	Ile359→Leu	Higher Km (defect)	6%
CYP2C19	Cryptic splice site in exon 5	No enzyme	10%
CYP2D6	Splice defect in in4/ex5 junction	No enzyme	23%
CYP2E1	Arg76→His	Less enzyme	<1%

part of chromosome 7p22. CYP3A5 has similar substrate specificity as CYP3A4 but appears to be expressed mainly in extrahepatic tissues in particularly the kidneys. It has a slower turnover for most substrates.

8.1.4   *Interindividual differences in drug metabolism*

The interindividual variation in expression of various forms of cytochrome P450 is extensive. In general the causes for this variability can be assigned to:

- genetic factors
- drug–drug interactions
- enzyme induction
- dietary factors/inhibition
- disease/inflammation

As a result, the hepatic expression of the different human drug metabolizing P450s differ from more than 20-fold, up to infinity (Shimada *et al.*, 1994). The enzyme which is the subject of the smallest variation appears to be CYP3A4, whereas those which are polymorphic of course exhibit the highest variation.

8.1.4.1.   *Genetic polymorphism of drug metabolizing P450s*

As mentioned, five of the drug metabolizing P450s are polymorphic (Table 8.3). Of those, the functionally important polymorphic alleles of *CYP2A6* and *CYP2E1* are rather rare, and therefore of less importance from a general point of

> The individual variation in expression of various forms of cytochrome P450 is extensive.

Table 8.4 Variant alleles of phase 1 and phase 2 drug metabolizing enzymes causing defective, partially defective, qualitatively altered or ultrarapid metabolism

Defective	Partially defective	Altered function	Ultraeffective
CYP2A6			
CYP2C9	CYP2C9	CYP2C9	
CYP2C19	CYP2C19		
CYP2D6	CYP2D6	CYP2D6	CYP2D6
	CYP2E1		
NAT-1			
NAT-2	NAT-2		
GSTM1			GSTM1
GSTT1			
UGT-1			

view, whereas the polymorphisms of *CYP2C9*, *CYP2C19* and *CYP2D6* are of great importance for drug metabolism and would have to be taken into consideration during drug development. Although only 2–3 different alleles have to be considered in the two first cases, the number of *CYP2D6* alleles is probably more than 50 (Marez *et al.*, 1997). For a more detailed overview of the polymorphic P450s, see Ingelman-Sundberg and Johansson (1995) and Ingelman-Sundberg (1997b).

Besides the P450 genes, it is clear that many of the phase 2 enzymes are also polymorphic. Defective alleles have been found encoding *N*-acetyltransferases, glutathione *S* transferases and UDP-glucuronosyltransferases. In addition, it has become evident that besides defective alleles, genes causing partially deficient, altered or ultrarapid drug metabolism are also polymorphically distributed (Table 8.4).

The ultrarapid metabolism is caused by the presence of multiple gene copies on one allele (Johansson *et al.*, 1993; McLellan *et al.*, 1997), whereas CYP2C9 (Rettie *et al.*, 1994) and CYP2D6 (Oscarson *et al.*, 1997) exist in variants with altered substrate specificities. In these cases, *in vitro* systems are of utmost importance for the characterization of the properties and the possible clinical consequences.

Besides the genetic aspects, also endogenous or exogenous factors influence the rate of drug metabolism within an individual.

8.1.4.2 *Pathophysiological conditions*

It is evident that disease might impair the capacity of the liver to metabolize drugs, an effect that is quantitatively important. Thus, a simple infection is known to cause down-regulation of several forms of hepatic P450, mainly due to the cytokine mediated decrease of gene expression (Morgan, 1997; Muntane *et al.*, 1995; Muntane-Relat *et al.*, 1995). Liver diseases like hepatitis, cirrhosis and liver cancer are known to impair the hepatic capacity for drug metabolism (George *et al.*, 1995).

8.1.4.3 Environmental factors

As evident from Table 8.1, most of the drug metabolizing P450s are inducible. Among the inducers are cigarette smoke (CYP1A2), ethanol (CYP2E1), rifampicin (CYP2C9/19, CYP3A4), phenytoin (CYP2C9, CYP3A4), phenobarbital (CYP3A4), omeprazole (CYP1A2) and dexamethasone (CYP3A4). Thus, those P450s mainly affected are CYP1A2, CYP2C9 and CYP3A4. Such induction might lead to a progressive drug tolerance and clinically affect the drug–drug interactions (see Ronis and Ingelman-Sundberg, 1998), as exemplified, for example, by the lack of effect of triazolam in patients taking rifampicin (Villikka *et al.*, 1997). However, compared to the interindividual variation in constitutive P450 expression, the extent of variation caused by a specific inducer appears to be rather limited as assessed by the detection of expression of specific P450 forms in human livers after known intake of inducers (Beaune *et al.*, 1997).

8.2 *In vitro* methods for prediction of human drug metabolism

As discussed above the most important aspects for prediction are the routes and rates of human metabolism of a particular NCE, i.e. which metabolites are formed, at what rate and by which enzymes. Incubations of NCEs with microsomes or S9 fractions is good as a first screening method. To determine enzyme specificity chemical inhibitors and/or inhibitory antibodies can be used. A complementary approach is to do correlation studies using so-called phenotyped microsomes, i.e. microsomes which have been characterized with respect to marker activities for the different enzymes. It is however in many cases difficult to differentiate between the different enzymes, and the availability of human-derived material is of course a limiting factor. For this purpose microsomes from cells expressing single enzymes are extremely useful to assess the specific metabolic activity of an enzyme. Complete kinetic analyses should be carried

Enzyme levels in microsomes from heterologous expression systems often are considerably higher than in human liver microsomes and do not reflect the relative abundance in the liver.

out, and K_m and V_{max} should be determined. It is not enough to determine metabolism at single saturating concentrations as the relative importance of low-affinity, high-capacity enzymes are then often overestimated. It should be noted that the enzyme levels in microsomes from heterologous expression systems often are considerably higher than in human liver microsomes and do not reflect the relative abundance in the liver. Therefore it is extremely important to correct for the actual liver levels, using e.g. the estimations from Shimada and co-workers (1994).

Recently many reports have described methods to estimate human *in vivo* pharmacokinetic data from *in vitro* metabolism data (Bertz and Granneman, 1997; Houston, 1994; Iwatsubo *et al.*, 1997; Obach *et al.*, 1997), based on different scaling factors. It appears that the intrinsic clearance (V_{max}/K_m from enzyme kinetic studies) is the best value for scaling (Houston, 1994; Iwatsubo *et al.*, 1997) and reasonable predictions of total body clearance can be obtained in many cases.

For prediction of drug–drug interactions it is important to determine the potential inhibition of DMEs by an NCE. In this context it should be noted that a drug can be an inhibitor of one enzyme, but be metabolized (at a low affinity) by another enzyme, e.g. the high-affinity CYP2D6 inhibitor quinidine, which is metabolized by CYP3A4 (Guengerich *et al.*, 1986). For determination of the enzyme specific inhibition of an NCE, the drug is incubated at various concentrations together with a marker drug for the enzyme (see Table 8.2). The apparent K_i is determined (Crespi and Penman, 1997), which is used in mathematical models to estimate the *in vivo* importance of the enzyme inhibition (von Moltke *et al.*, 1994a). To facilitate large-scale screening of enzyme inhibition, microtitre plate assays using fluorescent detection systems are being developed (Crespi *et al.*, 1997).

Of course all results from *in vitro* predictions must be confirmed in *in vivo* studies, and should be a guidance when designing these studies. If the NCE is mainly metabolized by CYP3A4, interaction studies with, for example, ketoconazole might be carried out, and if it is mainly metabolized by CYP2D6 or CYP2C19, panels of volunteers with different genotypes should be used.

Another important aspect is the potential cytotoxic, mutagenic or carcinogenic effect of an NCE and its metabolites. As discussed in detail elsewhere in this book, this has for many years been studied in various cellular systems, either in eukaryotic cells such as V79 or AHH-1 TK+/− or in prokaryotes such as *Salmonella typhimurium*. Because these systems are essentially deficient in DME activity, the NCEs have first been incubated with microsomes or S9 fractions and subsequently the incubation mixture has been exposed to the test system. Many metabolites are unstable and/or cannot pass membrane barriers, and it is therefore beneficial with an *in situ* toxicity system, where the DMEs are present within the target cells. So-called homotopic systems have therefore been developed where various DMEs are heterologously expressed in cells where these effects can be directly assessed.

8.3 Heterologous expression systems for drug metabolizing enzymes

8.3.1 General aspects

The development of modern molecular biology technologies has greatly facilitated the study of DMEs. Heterologous expression systems have been developed, and in principle unlimited amounts of enzyme can be obtained once a specific cDNA is cloned. These systems can be used to study an enzyme's substrate specificity and kinetic parameters, and also be used to assess the effect of specific amino acid exchanges on enzyme structure and stability, and to study intracellular trafficking. In addition it has been speculated that engineered enzymes (so-called 'designer P450s') can be developed which can be used as bioreactors to catalyze specific chemical reactions for instance in the production of pharmaceuticals or in bioremediation.

The system of choice should be easy to use and propagate at a low cost and yield high expression of functional enzymes in the native folding state. No, or low, background enzyme levels/activities should be present, and in addition the membrane-bound enzymes need a suitable environment mimicking the microsomal membranes. For P450s the NADPH cytochrome P450 reductase, and in some cases cytochrome b_5, should already be present or be co-expressed in the system. The systems of heterologuously expressed enzymes have to be characterized with respect to the background activity of the whole cell, the stability and level of expression of the drug metabolizing enzyme, the specificity of the expressed enzyme, and the kinetics of the enzyme.

This section describes the commonly used systems for heterologous expression of DMEs, and discuss the advantages and disadvantages for each of the systems. It will be focused on heterologous expression systems employed for

> The systems of heterologously expressed enzymes have to be characterized with respect to the background activity of the whole cell, the stability and level of expression of the drug metabolizing enzyme, the specificity of the expressed enzyme, and the kinetics of the enzyme.

cytochrome P450s, although heterologous expression of some of the other DME are also discussed. For more detailed descriptions of the various systems, the reader is referred to published review articles (Friedberg and Wolf, 1996; Gonzalez and Korzekwa, 1995; Guengerich and Parikh, 1997; Waterman, 1994, and references therein). The basic principles of heterologous expression are shown in Figure 8.1.

8.3.2 *Bacteria*

Escherichia coli has always been an attractive systems for heterologous expression of proteins, mostly because they are easy to manipulate and of low culturing costs. Until the early 1990s, expression of active cytochrome P450s in bacteria was considered to be impossible, but thanks to pioneering work by Barnes *et al.* (1991) and Larson *et al.* (1991), today essentially all drug metabolizing human P450s have been expressed at high levels in *E. coli* (Guengerich *et al.*, 1996a; Parikh *et al.*, 1997) and are usually incorporated into the *E. coli* membrane.

The cDNA for the enzyme to be expressed is cloned into an expression vector downstream of an efficient promoter and a ribosome-binding site, and especially the expression vector pCWori$^+$ (Muchmore *et al.*, 1989) has been very useful. To achieve high expression levels the 5′-end of the cDNA has however to be modified and often multiple variants have to be screened for expression levels. One successful approach has been to replace the N-terminal part of the P450 with the N-terminal from the bovine CYP17, which was the first P450 successfully expressed in *E. coli* (Barnes *et al.*, 1991). Some general guidelines are to introduce mutations to minimize the hairpin formation in the very 5′-part of the cDNA (Barnes, 1996). In addition the second codon should be replaced with GCT, encoding alanine, which has been shown to be present in proteins which are highly expressed in *E. coli* (Looman *et al.*, 1987). Alternatively, a bacterial leader sequence such as *ompA* or *pelB* can be attached to the N-terminal of the enzyme (Pritchard *et al.*, 1997). This leader sequence should be cleaved away after translation, but this is not always the case.

One major problem has been the lack of heme incorporation into the expressed enzyme, and sometimes only a fraction of the P450 is found as holoprotein, unless the heme precursor δ-aminolevulinic acid (δ-ALA) is added to the culture medium. This problem seems to be very enzyme-specific and to obtain heme-saturation of CYP2D6, addition of δ-ALA is a prerequisite (Gillam *et al.*, 1995; Kempf *et al.*, 1995).

Because *E. coli* is essentially deficient in the electron donor components needed for P450s, these enzymes must be supplemented with P450 reductase and in some cases cytochrome b_5. This is carried out with purified enzymes (Guengerich *et al.*, 1996b) which are reconstituted with these components and phospholipids. This is a tedious work and it has also been shown that some enzymes such as CYP3A4 are very sensitive to the correct environment, which has to be optimized in every case (Ingelman-Sundberg *et al.*, 1996). However, recent progress in the coexpression of P450s and the P450 reductase has created fully active systems. This can be achieved by using two different vectors, but bicistronic constructs where the cDNA for both the enzymes are cloned in tandem on the same plasmid have been a very useful approach (Blake *et al.*, 1996; Dong and Porter, 1996; Parikh *et al.*, 1997), which typically yields an approximately 1:1 ratio between P450 and P450 reductase. Such systems can be used directly to measure activity, either in intact cells or using membrane fractions (Blake *et al.*, 1996).

The soluble phase 2 enzyme families *N*-acetyltransferases, glutathione-*S*-transferases and sulphotransferases have been successfully expressed in *E. coli.* In some cases expression has been optimized by introduction of silent mutations in the 5′ part of the cDNA (Widersten *et al.*, 1996). In addition many of the DMEs have been expressed in *Salmonella typhimurium*, where a coupled system to study the activation of a substance by a DME to a genotoxic product can be obtained (Guengerich *et al.*, 1996a), using traditional endpoints such as reversion mutagenesis assay. Such systems have been designed using sulphotransferases (Glatt *et al.*, 1995), NATs (Grant *et al.*, 1992; Wild *et al.*, 1995), GSTs (Simula *et al.*, 1993) and a combination of CYP1A2 and NAT (Josephy *et al.*, 1995).

8.3.3 *Yeast*

Saccharomyces cerevisiae (baker's yeast) was the first heterologous expression system used for P450s (Oeda *et al.*, 1985), and since then most human P450s have been expressed in yeast (Imaoka *et al.*, 1996). Yeast is an attractive system, because it is easy to manipulate but still is a eukaryotic cell, which contains endoplasmatic reticulum and mitochondria. The intracellular sorting machinery seems to be highly conserved between yeast and mammalian cells, and heterologous P450 are incorporated into the ER membrane.

Yeast has low background levels of P450s, because only one yeast P450-gene is constitutively expressed, namely lanosterol-C14-demethylase, and this enzyme seems totally inactive towards xenobiotics. The normal heme synthesis in yeast seems however to be sufficient even for heterologous P450s, and high heme-saturation is normally obtained. In addition, yeast is naturally devoid of essentially all phase 2 enzymes.

Various vectors have been developed to increase P450 expression in yeast (Urban *et al.*, 1990). Depending on the application use, either constitutive or inducible promoters can be used. Inducible promoter responding to, for example, galactose, copper or phosphate, are in many cases preferred, so the P450 production can be separated from cell growth. Otherwise the construct might be genetically unstable, which could result in slower growth and selection against the multicopy plasmids. For heterologous expression in yeast no N-terminal modification of the P450 is necessary, however it is important to delete as much as possible of the 5′-non coding region, which otherwise will decrease the level of expression (Pompon, 1988).

Although the yeast's P450 reductase gene CPR is constitutively expressed, it has been shown that it sometimes couples very poorly to the human P450s, especially to CYP3A4 (Peyronneau *et al.*, 1992), and the yeast cytochrome b_5 is unsuitable to donate electrons to the human enzyme. Three generations of yeast strains have therefore been developed, where the redox environment has been optimized by genetic manipulation of the yeast genome; the genes encoding P450 reductase and cytochrome b_5 have been replaced with the human counterparts, and are also under the control of a galactose-inducible promoter (Pompon *et al.*, 1996; Urban *et al.*, 1994). The enhancement of the P450-dependent activity by these optimized backgrounds is enzyme- and substrate-dependent, but can be as high as 73-fold, as for CYP3A4-mediated testosterone 6β-hydroxylation (Truan *et al.*, 1993). In addition, phase 2 enzymes such as epoxide hydrolase can be co-expressed, and thereby complete metabolic pathways can be generated (Gautier *et al.*, 1996).

8.3.4 *Insect cells*

The baculovirus expression system is an eukaryotic system which yields very high expression levels for many human enzymes, and typically 300–1000 pmol enzyme/mg cell lysate can be achieved for many of the P450s (Gonzalez *et al.*, 1991b). This group of viruses consists of more than 500 species, which can only infect insect cells, and for heterologous expression the AcMNPV virus is normally used. The virus has a lytic life-cycle and thus only transient expression can be achieved. Because the virus has a large genome of ≈130,000 bp, normal molecular biology techniques cannot be used, and special transfer-vectors have to be used for cloning.

The enzyme is expressed in insect Sf9 cells, which resemble mammalian cells in that they contain both endoplasmatic reticulum and mitochondria. They are, however, deficient in all electron-transport components needed for P450 activity, so this has to be added to accomplish an active system. Alternatively the P450 reductase and also cytochrome b_5 can be co-expressed in the same cell (Chen *et al.*, 1997; Lee *et al.*, 1996).

One problem is that the heme-incorporation is variable (50–90%), which can be significantly increased by addition of hemin to the culture medium. Many of the post-translational mechanisms are similar to mammalian cells, and CYP19A1 is for instance glycosylated as expected (Shimozawa *et al.*, 1993). This makes this system useful for UDP-glucuronosyl transferases, which need post-translational processing to be active (Nguyen and Tukey, 1997).

Because the cells are killed by the lytic virus after 2–3 days, this system cannot be used for long-term toxicity studies. There are however reports where it has been used as an *in situ* toxicity system for short-term treatments (Grant *et al.*, 1996).

8.3.5 *Mammalian cells*

8.3.5.1 *Transient expression*

COS-1 cells   The first mammalian cells used for heterologous expression of P450s was the COS-1 cell line (Zuber *et al.*, 1986). This cell line was selected from African green monkey kidney fibroblast CV-1 cells, which had been transformed with SV40 (Gluzman, 1981). Because these cells originate from kidney, which is involved in the metabolism of vitamin D by P450s in both the endoplasmatic reticulum and the mitochondria, they express the reducing enzymes for both these compartments, although at low levels.

The cells express the SV40 T antigen which is required for viral replication. Thus, all expression vectors with the SV40 origin of replication will also replicate in these cells. The most commonly used vector is the pCMV series (Andersson *et al.*, 1989; Clark and Waterman, 1991), which are transfected to the cells with standard methods such as

Figure 8.2

The cDNA which is to be expressed is cloned in front of an artificial promoter in a vector suitable for the type of cells which is going to be used (A). The vector contains sequences for replication in the cell, and for initiation and termination of transcription, as well as a gene encoding resistance to a drug which will be used for selection and maintenance of the plasmid within the cell. After transfection/transformation to the host cell (B), plasmids replicate and expression of the cDNA is initiated (C). Transformants are selected and cultured in appropriate medium. The cells can subsequently be harvested and microsomes can be isolated, alternatively many cell types containing fully active systems can be directly used for metabolism studies. It should however be noted that all these enzymes are individuals, and each system has to be optimized for each specific enzyme.

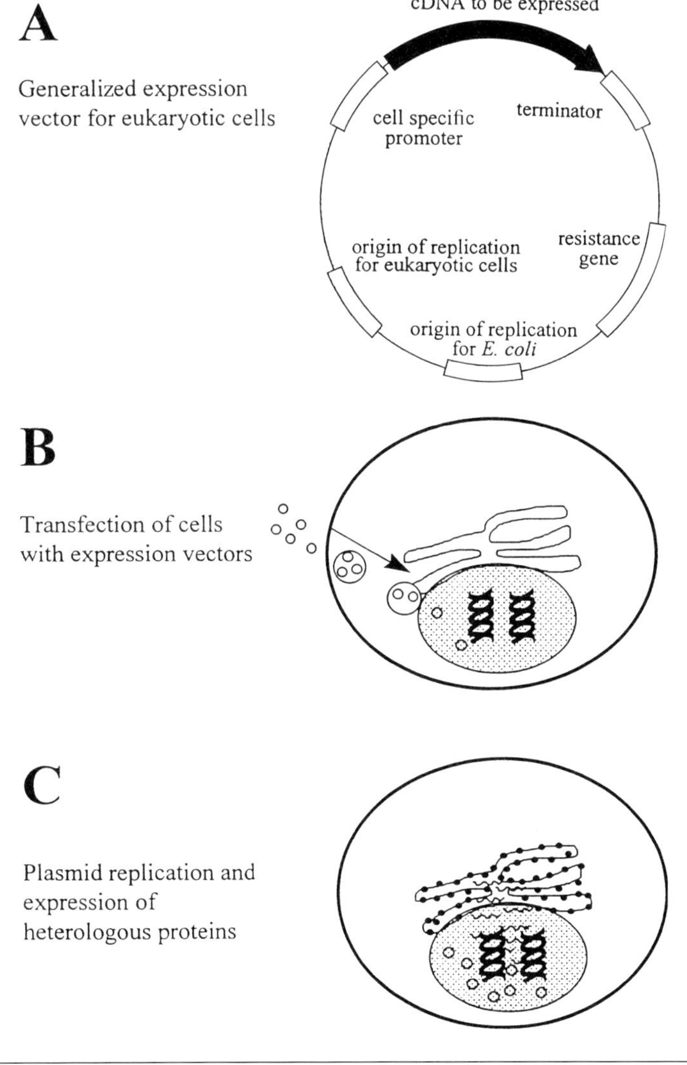

A
Generalized expression
vector for eukaryotic cells

cDNA to be expressed
cell specific promoter
terminator
origin of replication for eukaryotic cells
resistance gene
origin of replication for E. coli

B
Transfection of cells
with expression vectors

C
Plasmid replication and
expression of
heterologous proteins

transfection with DEAE-dextran, calcium phosphate precipitation, liposomes or electroporation. These vectors contain a strong human cytomegalovirus promoter, but the total expression levels are still relatively low mostly because of the relatively low transfection efficiency (Clark and Waterman, 1991). The vectors replicate in the cells and start to express P450 with peak expression levels after 2 to 3 days, after which the levels decline rapidly.

Because of the low expression levels, no P450-spectra can be obtained, and the system is not practically suitable for large-scale screening of metabolism. Its major use has been in screening for activities of newly cloned cDNAs and to study the effect of amino acid exchanges on enzyme activity, mainly because it is easy to clone and mutate the cDNAs, and there is no need to modify 5' and 3' flanking regions. Several cDNAs can be co-transfected and thereby complete metabolic pathways can be generated.

Vaccinia virus-mediated expression For certain applications it is useful to achieve high level expression in hepatoma cell lines, and for this purpose a vaccinia virus can be used in, for example, HepG2 cells (Gonzalez, 1993; Gonzalez *et al.*, 1991a). The vaccinia virus is a lytic virus with a genome of approximately 187,000 bp and can infect any mammalian cell. As with baculovirus, this size of the genome makes cloning and modification impossible with normal molecular biology techniques, and special transfer vectors are needed. There are also some safety concerns when working with this attenuated derivative of a cow pox virus.

For expression of cytochrome P450s no modifications are needed in the 5' and 3' flanking regions and relatively high expression levels can normally be achieved. Because the hepatoma cell line HepG2 contains both P450 reductase and cytochrome b_5, active functional systems can be obtained without addition or co-expression of any other components.

8.3.5.2 Stable expression

Human B lymphoblastoid cell line AHH TK+/− The human B lymphoblastoid cell line AHH TK+/− has been extensively utilized for stable expression of human P450s in mammalian cells (Crespi *et al.*, 1993). This cell line is a derivative of the RPMI 1788 cell line, which is easy to handle, and can be grown in suspension with medium supplemented with donor horse serum instead of the more expensive fetal bovine serum used for most other cell lines. It has a stable, near-diploid chromosome number, and because it is heterozygous at the thymidine kinase (TK) locus, it is especially suitable for gene locus mutation assays. As the name implies, the cell line contains some basal P450 activity, however these activities are very low, and barely above the limit of detection.

Vectors based on sequences from the Epstein Barr virus is used, and the expression is controlled by a promoter from the herpes simplex virus thymidine kinase gene. The cells are transfected and positive clones are selected and maintained through resistance to either hygromycin B or 1-histidinol, yielding stable expression levels of up to 200 pmol/mg microsomal protein. Using different vectors, multiple cDNAs can be co-expressed in the cell lines. The catalytic activity of the P450s can be enhanced by co-expression of P450 reductase, and in some cases also cytochrome b_5 (Crespi and Penman, 1997). Other DMEs such as epoxide hydrolase, UDP-glucuronosyl transferases and flavin-containing mono-oxygenases have also been successfully expressed in AHH-1 TK +/− cells.

As mentioned above the cells are especially useful for toxicological studies (Langenbach *et al.*, 1992), as *in situ* toxicity systems. Mutagenicity can be examined as chromosomal aberrations, and gene locus mutation assays at the hypoxanthine guanine phosphoribosyl transferase and thymidine kinase loci.

V79 cells The V79 Chinese hamster cells have a widespread use in genetic toxicology and mutagenesis research, where studies are carried out with biological endpoints such as cell viability, cytotoxicity, mutagenicity, chromosomal aberration and micronucleus formation (Bradley *et al.*, 1981). Because they are deficient in P450 expression it has been difficult to assess the effect of chemicals which need metabolic activation to exert their toxicity.

Methods have been developed to stably express various P450s in the V79 cells (Doehmer and Oesch, 1991; Doehmer *et al.*, 1995), where the P450 in cloned into an expression vector and subsequently spontaneously integrated into the genome. Positive clones are selected, and assayed for P450 expression and the corresponding activity. The expression levels are usually relatively low, but functional systems can be obtained because the cells contain both P450 reductase and cytochrome b_5, albeit at low levels. Recent studies have shown that the activity can be increased by co-expression of P450 reductase (Schneider *et al.*, 1996).

Because of the relatively low expression levels and expensive culturing conditions, these cells are of low value for the screening of drug metabolism. However, they constitute a useful tool for screening of cytotoxicity and mutagenicity by NCEs and their metabolites.

Because of the relatively low expression levels and expensive culturing conditions, V79 cells are of low value for the screening of drug metabolism. However, they constitute a useful tool for screening of cytotoxicity and mutagenicity by NCEs and their metabolites.

8.3.6 *Utility for drug screening – a comparison*

The cDNA expressed human P450s in microsomes provides an important tool in the identification of the form of P450 being responsible for the phase 1 metabolism of a particular NCE or drug. In combination with data obtained from incubations using various relatively specific inhibitors of human P450s, quite unequivocal results can be obtained concerning enzyme specificity, metabolite pattern and rate of P450 dependent oxidation, with possibilities to extrapolate the specific contribution by the enzyme to the *in vivo* situation (cf. Kobayashi *et al.*, 1997; Kudo *et al.*, 1997; Olesen and Linnet, 1997; Rochat *et al.*, 1997; von Moltke *et al.*, 1997). In particular, microsomes containing specific P450s from cDNA expression in human B-lymphoblastoid cells have received much application. The number of companies supplying microsomes from P450 cDNA expressing cells is now rapidly growing. Hitherto, microsomes derived from yeast cells and bacteria have received less attention, perhaps because of their lower commercial availability.

In our laboratory we have within the EU-supported EUROCYP project expressed most drug metabolizing P450s in yeast, based on the methods described by Urban *et al.* (1990) and Gautier *et al.* (1993) using the galactose driven promoter, with good results. The expression levels vary between 30 and 150 pmol per mg of protein and all P450s are catalytically active. This expression resembles, from quantitative aspects, that seen in human microsomes and such preparations are well suited for studies of enzyme selectivity and turnover rates. The transfected yeast cells are stable in the cold for years and could easily be fermented for enzyme production. As experienced up to now, the kinetic properties of the yeast preparations of the different P450s are very similar to those in intact human liver microsomes. Similar good experience has also been seen by other investigators (Imaoka *et al.*, 1996).

The major advantage with bacterial expression is the amount of enzyme that can be obtained (cf. Friedberg and Wolf, 1996; Parikh *et al.*, 1997). This makes the bacterial system of great importance for production of large amounts of P450 that can be used for structural and extensive kinetic studies, mainly of purified enzyme preparations properly reconstituted. For production of large amounts of metabolites to be identified from the NCEs, this system evidently has major advantages. Recent results imply the possibility to use whole cell incubation systems for the examination of P450 dependent drug metabolism in cells also containing P450 reductase (Parikh *et al.*, 1997). The permeability properties of the bacterial cell wall is however expected to exclude the use of this system for larger and more polar compounds. The question might be raised whether isolated bacterial membranes are well suited for studies of NCE metabolism. Although being well incorporated into the membrane, the relative levels of the P450s is very high and the bacterial membrane is different from that of human liver microsomes which might be a problem when examining the right kinetic properties of the P450 dependent drug metabolism. However, no thorough comparative study exist that has addressed this problem in detail.

Another problem with the bacterial expression system is, according to our own experience, that certain polymorphic forms of P450s appear not to be properly folded, yielding catalytically inactive enzyme products, as compared to results obtained using similar expression in either yeast or COS-1 cells. This might be due to differences in the nature of chaperones or other proteins necessary for the correct enzyme synthesis.

The different expression systems exhibit somewhat different properties with respect to the functional environment of the enzymes. Thus, the microsomes from various types of cells differ in their lipid compositions and, thus, also in their rigidity. Such factors might be of importance for reconstitution of, for example, CYP1A2 and CYP3A4 dependent catalytic activities using specific substrates (Ingelman-Sundberg *et al.*, 1996; Yun *et al.*, 1997). Furthermore the ratio between the P450 reductase and P450 differs in the various systems and this is a factor that might be of importance in special cases, e.g. for reconstitution of the R144C variant of CYP2C9, where this amino acid change is known to influence the affinity of the hemoprotein for the P450 reductase and the relative rate of product formation, as compared to the wildtype enzyme (Crespi and Miller, 1997).

Expression of CYP3A4 represents an important application of the heterologous systems. In Table 8.5, we have compared the CYP3A4 expression levels and catalytic activities obtained using the different heterologous systems described. As expected, the bacterial expression systems yield the highest expression level per litre of culture, whereas the highest specific membranous content of CYP3A4 has been seen in the baculovirus Sf9 insect cell system. High turnover values for CYP3A4-dependent testosterone 6β-hydroxylation is observed in systems with human P450 reductase co-expressed using both the insect cells and bacteria, although in yeast, in the published reports there seems to have been an

Table 8.5　A comparison of CYP3A4 expression in various heterologous expression systems

Expression system	Expression level (nmol/l)	Specific content (pmol/mg)	Activity testosterone 6β-hydroxylation (min⁻¹)	Incubation conditions	References
E. coli	200–370	220–330	6	reconstituted with reductase + b_5 + GSH	Gillam *et al.*, 1993
E. coli			23	reconstituted with reductase + b_5 + GSH	Ingelman-Sundberg *et al.*, 1996
E. coli	200	215	17.3–25.5	reductase co-expressed	Blake *et al.*, 1996
E. coli	230		6.3–14	reductase co-expressed	Parikh *et al.*, 1997
S. cerevisiae		156	4.7	reconstituted with reductase + b_5	Imaoka *et al.*, 1996
S. cerevisiae	5–10	50–150	0.04	native reductase	Peyronneau *et al.*, 1992
			1.0	yeast reductase overexpressed	
			0.2	b_5 co-expressed	
			1.2	b_5 co-expressed + yeast reductase overexpressed	
Baculovirus/Sf9	103	459	24.8	reconstituted with reductase + b_5	Buters *et al.*, 1994
Baculovirus/Sf9		51–53	27.3	reductase co-expressed	Lee *et al.*, 1995
Baculovirus/T. ni		107–235	66.6	reductase co-expressed	Lee *et al.*, 1995
AHH TK+/−		300	15	native background	Crespi and Penman, 1997
AHH TK+/−			44	reductase co-expressed	
V79		6[a]	16–39[a]	reductase co-expressed	Schneider *et al.*, 1996
Vacciniavirus/HepG2		75	15	native background	Aoyama *et al.*, 1989
Vacciniavirus/HepG2			29.6	native background	Buters *et al.*, 1994

[a] based on immunochemical quantification
b_5, cytochrome b_5
GSH, glutathione

We would expect the rapid development of an increasing number of systems where the different human P450s are heterologously expressed at a high efficiency. There will be, however, a lot of work to characterize these systems with respect to proper function and substrate specificities in comparison to the situation in native human liver microsomes.

The results obtained are of high importance during the drug development process, and makes the process cheaper and more efficient.

inproductive coupling between the yeast reductase and CYP3A4 with very low rates of CYP3A4 dependent catalytic reactions.

In conclusion, we would expect the rapid development of an increasing number of systems where the different human P450s are heterologously expressed at a higher efficiency. There will be, however, a lot of work to characterize these systems with respect to proper function and substrate specificities in comparison to the situation in native human liver microsomes. In particular these problems might be most accentuated with polymorphic variants of the different P450s that exhibit reduced but not abolished enzyme activities. At the present time, however, the possibility to use microsomes from cDNA expressing mammalian and insect cells containing the important drug metabolizing human wild type P450s provides a most useful and appropriate tool for studying metabolic pathways, enzyme selectivities and rates of metabolism exerted by these hemoproteins. The results obtained are of high importance during the drug development process, and makes the process cheaper and more efficient.

Acknowledgements

We are indebted to Mrs AnnCatrin Brattström for valuable aid during the preparation of this manuscript. The research in the authors' laboratory is supported by grants from EU (Biomed 2), The Swedish Medical Research Council and from Astra AB.

References

Andersson, S., Davis, D.L., Dahlbäck, H., Jörnvall, H. and Russell, D.W., 1989, Cloning, structure, and expression of the mitochondrial cytochrome P-450 sterol 26-hydroxylase, a bile acid biosynthetic enzyme, *J Biol Chem*, **264**, 8222–8229.

Aoyama, T., Yamano, S., Waxman, D.J., Lapenson, D.P., Meyer, U.A., Fischer, V. *et al.*, 1989, Cytochrome P-450 hPCN3, a novel cytochrome P-450 IIIA gene product that is differentially expressed in adult human liver. cDNA and deduced amino acid sequence and distinct specificities of cDNA-expressed hPCN1 and hPCN3 for the metabolism of steroid hormones and cyclosporine, *J Biol Chem*, **264**, 10388–10395.

Barnes, H.J., 1996, Maximizing expression of eukaryotic cytochrome P450s in *Escherichia coli, Methods Enzymol*, **272**, 3–14.

Barnes, H.J., Arlotto, M.P. and Waterman, M.R., 1991, Expression and enzymatic activity of recombinant cytochrome P450 17 alpha-hydroxylase in *Escherichia coli, Proc Natl Acad Sci USA*, **88**, 5597–5601.

Beaune, P., DeWaziers, I., Gervot, L., Belloc, C., Perrot, N., Barouki, R. *et al.*, 1997, Induction of Human P450s in vitro, in Sundvall, A., Alván, G., Lindgren, E., Moldéus, P., Salomonsson, T. and Sjöberg, P. (eds) *The use of Human In Vitro systems to support preclinical and clinical safety assessment*, vol. 197, pp. 35–40; The Swedish Association of the Pharmaceutical Industry and Medical Products Agency.

Bertz, R.J. and Granneman, G.R., 1997, Use of in vitro and in vivo data to estimate the likelihood of metabolic pharmacokinetic interactions, *Clin Pharmacokinet*, **32**, 210–258.

Blake, J.A., Pritchard, M., Ding, S., Smith, G.C., Burchell, B., Wolf, C.R. *et al.*, 1996, Coexpression of a human P450 (CYP3A4) and P450 reductase generates a highly functional monooxygenase system in *Escherichia coli, FEBS Lett*, **397**, 210–214.

Bradley, M.O., Bhuyan, B., Francis, M.C., Langenbach, R., Peterson, A. and Huberman, E., 1981, Mutagenesis by chemical agents in V79 chinese hamster cells: a review and analysis of the literature. A report of the Gene-Tox Program, *Mutat Res*, **87**, 81–142.

Buters, J.T., Korzekwa, K.R., Kunze, K.L., Omata, Y., Hardwick, J.P. and Gonzalez, F.J., 1994, cDNA-directed expression of human cytochrome P450 CYP3A4 using baculovirus, *Drug Metab Dispos*, **22**, 688–692.

Chen, L., Buters, J.T., Hardwick, J.P., Tamura, S., Penman, B.W., Gonzalez, F.J. *et al.*, 1997, Coexpression of cytochrome P4502A6 and human NADPH-P450 oxidoreductase in the baculovirus system, *Drug Metab Dispos*, **25**, 399–405.

Clark, B.J. and Waterman, M.R., 1991, Heterologous expression of mammalian P450 in COS cells, *Methods Enzymol*, **206**, 100–108.

Crespi, C.L., Langenbach, R. and Penman, B.W., 1993, Human cell lines, derived from AHH-1 TK+/− human lymphoblasts, genetically engineered for expression of cytochromes P450, *Toxicology*, **82**, 89–104.

Crespi, C.L. and Miller, V.P., 1997, The R144C change in the CYP2C9*2 allele alters interaction of the cytochrome P450 with NADPH:cytochrome P450 oxidoreductase, *Pharmacogenetics*, **7**, 203–210.

Crespi, C.L., Miller, V.P. and Penman, B.W., 1997, Microtiter plate assays for inhibition of human, drug-metabolizing cytochromes P450, *Anal Biochem*, **248**, 188–190.

Crespi, C.L. and Penman, B.W., 1997, Use of cDNA-expressed human cytochrome P450 enzymes to study potential drug–drug interactions, *Adv Pharmacol*, **43**, 171–188.

Doehmer, J. and Oesch, F., 1991, V79 Chinese hamster cells genetically engineered for stable expression of cytochromes P450, *Methods Enzymol*, **206**, 117–123.

Doehmer, J., Schneider, A., Fassbender, M., Soballa, V., Schmalix, W.A. and Greim, H., 1995, Genetically engineered mammalian cells and applications, *Toxicol Lett*, **82–83**, 823–827.

Dong, J. and Porter, T.D., 1996, Coexpression of mammalian cytochrome P450 and reductase in *Escherichia coli, Arch Biochem Biophys*, **327**, 254–259.

FDA, 1997, *Guidance for Industry – Drug Metabolism/ Drug Interaction Studies in the Drug Development Process: Studies In Vitro*. Rockville, MD: Department of Health and Human Services, U. S. Food and Drug Administration.

Fernandez-Salguero, P., Hoffman, S.M., Cholerton, S., Mohrenweiser, H., Raunio, H., Rautio, A. *et al.*, 1995, A genetic polymorphism in coumarin 7-hydroxylation: sequence of the human CYP2A genes and identification of variant CYP2A6 alleles, *Am J Hum Genet*, **57**, 651–660.

Friedberg, T. and Wolf, C.R., 1996, Recombinant DNA technology as an investigative tool in drug metabolism research, *Adv Drug Deliv Rev*, **22**, 187–213.

Gautier, J.C., Lecoeur, S., Cosme, J., Perret, A., Urban, P., Beaune, P. *et al.*, 1996, Contribution of human cytochrome P450 to benzo[a]pyrene and benzo[a]pyrene-7,8-dihydrodiol metabolism, as predicted from heterologous expression in yeast, *Pharmacogenetics*, **6**, 489–499.

Gautier, J.C., Urban, P., Beaune, P. and Pompon, D., 1993, Engineered yeast cells as model to study coupling between human xenobiotic metabolizing enzymes. Simulation of the two first steps of benzo[a]pyrene activation, *Eur J Biochem*, **211**, 63–72.

Gebhardt, A.C., Lucas, D., Menez, J.F. and Seitz, H.K., 1997, Chlormethiazole inhibition of cytochrome P450 2E1 as assessed by chlorzoxazone hydroxylation in humans, *Hepatology*, **26**, 957–961.

George, J., Murray, M., Byth, K. and Farrell, G.C., 1995, Differential alterations of cytochrome P450 proteins in livers from patients with severe chronic liver disease, *Hepatology*, **21**, 120–128.

Gillam, E.M., Baba, T., Kim, B.R., Ohmori, S. and Guengerich, F.P., 1993, Expression of modified human cytochrome P450 3A4 in *Escherichia coli* and purification and reconstitution of the enzyme, *Arch Biochem Biophys*, **305**, 123–131.

Gillam, E.M., Guo, Z., Martin, M.V., Jenkins, C.M. and Guengerich, F.P., 1995, Expression of cytochrome P450 2D6 in *Escherichia coli*, purification, and spectral and catalytic characterization, *Arch Biochem Biophys*, **319**, 540–550.

Glatt, H., Bartsch, I., Czich, A., Seidel, A. and Falany, C.N., 1995, *Salmonella* strains and mammalian cells genetically engineered for expression of sulfotransferases, *Toxicol Lett*, **82–83**, 829–834.

Gluzman, Y., 1981, SV40-transformed simian cells support the replication of early SV40 mutants, *Cell*, **23**, 175–182.

Gonzalez, F.J., 1993, Molecular biology of human xenobiotic-metabolizing cytochromes P450: role of vaccinia virus cDNA expression in evaluating catalytic function, *Toxicology*, **82**, 77–88.

Gonzalez, F.J., Aoyama, T. and Gelboin, H.V., 1991a, Expression of mammalian cytochrome P450 using vaccinia virus, *Methods Enzymol*, **206**, 85–92.

Gonzalez, F.J., Kimura, S., Tamura, S. and Gelboin, H.V., 1991b, Expression of mammalian cytochrome P450 using baculovirus, *Methods Enzymol*, **206**, 93–99.

Gonzalez, F.J. and Korzekwa, K.R., 1995, Cytochromes P450 expression systems, *Annu Rev Pharmacol Toxicol*, **35**, 369–390.

Grant, D.F., Greene, J.F., Pinot, F., Borhan, B., Moghaddam, M.F., Hammock, B.D. *et al.*, 1996, Development of an *in situ* toxicity assay system using recombinant baculoviruses, *Biochem Pharmacol*, **51**, 503–515.

Grant, D.M., Josephy, P.D., Lord, H.L. and Morrison, L.D., 1992, *Salmonella typhimurium* strains expressing human arylamine N-acetyltransferases: metabolism and mutagenic activation of aromatic amines, *Cancer Res*, **52**, 3961–3964.

Guengerich, F.P., Gillam, E.M. and Shimada, T., 1996a, New applications of bacterial systems to problems in toxicology, *Crit Rev Toxicol*, **26**, 551–583.

Guengerich, F.P., Martin, M.V., Guo, Z. and Chun, Y.J., 1996b, Purification of functional recombinant P450s from bacteria, *Methods Enzymol*, **272**, 35–44.

Guengerich, F.P., Muller-Enoch, D. and Blair, I.A., 1986, Oxidation of quinidine by human liver cytochrome P-450, *Mol Pharmacol*, **30**, 287–295.

Guengerich, F.P. and Parikh, A., 1997, Expression of drug-metabolizing enzymes, *Curr Opin Biotechnol*, **8**, 623–628.

Houston, J.B., 1994, Utility of in vitro drug metabolism data in predicting in vivo metabolic clearance, *Biochem Pharmacol*, **47**, 1469–1479.

Hu, Y., Oscarson, M., Johansson, I., Yue, Q.Y., Dahl, M.L., Tabone, M. *et al.*, 1997, Genetic polymorphism of human *CYP2E1*: characterization of two variant alleles, *Mol Pharmacol*, **51**, 370–376.

Imaoka, S., Yamada, T., Hiroi, T., Hayashi, K., Sakaki, T., Yabusaki, Y. *et al.*, 1996, Multiple forms of human P450 expressed in *Saccharomyces cerevisiae*. Systematic characterization and comparison with those of the rat, *Biochem Pharmacol*, **51**, 1041–1050.

Ingelman-Sundberg, M., 1997a, The Gerhard Zbinden Memorial Lecture. Genetic polymorphism of drug metabolizing enzymes. Implications for toxicity of drugs and other xenobiotics, *Arch Toxicol Suppl*, **19**, 3–13.

Ingelman-Sundberg, M., 1997b, Major human cytochromes P450 in xenobiotic metabolism, in Sundwall, A., Alván, G., Lindgren, E., Moldéus, P., Salomonsson, T. and Sjöberg, P. (eds) *The use of human In Vitro systems to support preclinical and clinical safety assessment*, pp. 5–12, The Swedish Association on the Pharmaceutical Industry & Medical Products Agency.

Ingelman-Sundberg, M., Hagbjörk, A.-L., Ueng, Y.F., Yamazaki, H. and Guengerich, F.P., 1996, High rates of substrate hydroxylation by human cytochrome P450 3A4 in reconstituted membranous vesicles: influence of membrane charge, *Biochem Biophys Res Commun*, **221**, 318–322.

Ingelman-Sundberg, M. and Johansson, I., 1995, The molecular genetics of the human drug metabolizing cytochrome P450s, in Pacifici, G. and Fracchia, G.N. (eds) *Advances in Drug metabolism in Man*, vol. EUR 15439 EN, EC, DGXII-E-4, ECSC-EC-EAEC, pp. 543–586, Luxembourg: Office for Official Publications of the European Communities.

Iwatsubo, T., Hirota, N., Ooie, T., Suzuki, H., Shimada, N., Chiba, K. *et al.*, 1997, Prediction of in vivo drug metabolism in the human liver from in vitro metabolism data, *Pharmacol Ther*, **73**, 147–171.

Johansson, I., Lundqvist, E., Bertilsson, L., Dahl, M.L., Sjöqvist, F. and Ingelman-Sundberg, M., 1993, Inherited amplification of an active gene in the cytochrome P450 CYP2D locus as a cause of ultrarapid metabolism of debrisoquine, *Proc Natl Acad Sci USA*, **90**, 11825–11829.

Josephy, P.D., DeBruin, L.S., Lord, H.L., Oak, J.N., Evans, D.H., Guo, Z. *et al.*, 1995, Bioactivation of aromatic amines by recombinant human cytochrome P4501A2 expressed in Ames tester strain bacteria: a substitute for activation by mammalian tissue preparations, *Cancer Res*, **55**, 799–802.

Kempf, A.C., Zanger, U.M. and Meyer, U.A., 1995, Truncated human P450 2D6: expression in *Escherichia coli*, Ni^{2+}-chelate affinity purification, and characterization of solubility and aggregation, *Arch Biochem Biophys*, **321**, 277–288.

Kobayashi, K., Chiba, K., Yagi, T., Shimada, N., Taniguchi, T., Horie, T. *et al.*, 1997, Identification of cytochrome P450 isoforms involved in citalopram N-demethylation by human liver microsomes, *J Pharmacol Exp Ther*, **280**, 927–933.

Kudo, S., Uchida, M. and Odomi, M., 1997, Metabolism of carteolol by cDNA-expressed human cytochrome P450, *Eur J Clin Pharmacol*, **52**, 479–485.

Langenbach, R., Smith, P.B. and Crespi, C., 1992, Recombinant DNA approaches for the development of metabolic systems used in in vitro toxicology, *Mutat Res*, **277**, 251–275.

Larson, J., Coon, M. and Porter, T., 1991, Alcohol-inducible cytochrome P450IIE1 lacking the hydrophobic NH$_2$-terminal segment retains catalytic activity and is membrane-bound when expressed in *Escherichia coli*, *J Biol Chem*, **266**, 7321–7324.

Lee, C.A., Kadwell, S.H., Kost, T.A. and Serabjit-Singh, C.J., 1995, CYP3A4 expressed by insect cells infected with a recombinant baculovirus containing both CYP3A4 and human NADPH-cytochrome P450 reductase is catalytically similar to human liver microsomal CYP3A4, *Arch Biochem Biophys*, **319**, 157–167.

Lee, C.A., Kost, T.A. and Serabjit-Singh, C.J., 1996, Recombinant baculovirus strategy for coexpression of functional human cytochrome P450 and P450 reductase, *Methods Enzymol*, **272**, 86–95.

Li, A.P. (ed.), 1997, *Drug-drug interactions: scientific and regulatory perspectives*, Advances in pharmacology, San Diego: Academic Press.

Looman, A.C., Bodlaender, J., Comstock, L.J., Eaton, D., Jhurani, P., de Boer, H.A. *et al.*, 1987, Influence of the codon following the AUG initiation codon on the expression of a modified lacZ gene in *Escherichia coli*, *EMBO J*, **6**, 2489–2492.

Marez, D., Legrand, M., Sabbagh, N., Guidice, J.M., Spire, C., Lafitte, J.J. *et al.*, 1997, Polymorphism of the cytochrome P450 CYP2D6 gene in a European population:

characterization of 48 mutations and 53 alleles, their frequencies and evolution, *Pharmacogenetics*, **7**, 193–202.

McLellan, R.A., Oscarson, M., Seidegard, J., Evans, D.A. and Ingelman-Sundberg, M., 1997, Frequent occurrence of CYP2D6 gene duplication in Saudi Arabians, *Pharmacogenetics*, **7**, 187–191.

Monro, A.M., 1996, Why do so many drugs fail between the laboratory and the marketplace?, in Sundwall, A., Alván, G., Lindgren, E., Moldéus, P., Salmonsson, T. and Sjöberg, P. (eds) *The Use of Human In Vitro System to Support Preclinical and Clinical Safety Assessment*, pp. 1–4, Stockholm, Sweden: The Swedish Association of the Pharmaceutical Industry and Medical Products Agency.

Morgan, E.T., 1997, Regulation of cytochromes P450 during inflammation and infection, *Drug Metab Rev*, **29**, 1129–1188.

Muchmore, D.C., McIntosh, L.P., Russell, C.B., Anderson, D.E. and Dahlquist, F.W., 1989, Expression and nitrogen-15 labeling of proteins for proton and nitrogen-15 nuclear magnetic resonance, *Methods Enzymol*, **177**, 44–73.

Muntane, J., Longo, V., Mitjavila, M.T., Gervasi, P.G. and Ingelman-Sundberg, M., 1995, Effect of carrageenan-induced granuloma on hepatic cytochrome P-450 isozymes in rats, *Inflammation*, **19**, 143–156.

Muntane-Relat, J., Ourlin, J.C., Domergue, J. and Maurel, P., 1995, Differential effects of cytokines on the inducible expression of CYP1A1, CYP1A2, and CYP3A4 in human hepatocytes in primary culture, *Hepatology*, **22**, 1143–1153.

Nguyen, N. and Tukey, R.H., 1997, Baculovirus-directed expression of rabbit UDP-glucuronosyltransferases in *Spodoptera frugiperda* cells, *Drug Metab Dispos*, **25**, 745–749.

Obach, R.S., Baxter, J.G., Liston, T.E., Silber, B.M., Jones, B.C., MacIntyre, F. *et al.*, 1997, The prediction of human pharmacokinetic parameters from preclinical and in vitro metabolism data, *J Pharmacol Exp Ther*, **283**, 46–58.

Oeda, K., Sakaki, T. and Ohkawa, H., 1985, Expression of rat liver cytochrome P-450MC cDNA in *Saccharomyces cerevisiae*, *DNA*, **4**, 203–210.

Olesen, O.V. and Linnet, K., 1997, Hydroxylation and demethylation of the tricyclic antidepressant nortriptyline by cDNA-expressed human cytochrome P-450 isozymes, *Drug Metab Dispos*, **25**, 740–744.

Oscarson, M., Hidestrand, M., Johansson, I. and Ingelman-Sundberg, M., 1997, A combination of mutations in the *CYP2D6*17* (*CYP2D6Z*) allele causes alterations in enzyme function, *Mol Pharmacol*, **52**, 1034–1040.

Parikh, A., Gillam, E.M. and Guengerich, F.P., 1997, Drug metabolism by *Escherichia coli* expressing human cytochromes P450, *Nat Biotechnol*, **15**, 784–788.

Parkinson, A., 1996, Biotransformation of xenobiotics, in Klaasen, C.D. (ed.) *Casarett and Doull's toxicology: the basic science of poisons*, pp. 113–186, New York: McGraw-Hill.

Peyronneau, M.A., Renaud, J.P., Truan, G., Urban, P., Pompon, D. and Mansuy, D., 1992, Optimization of yeast-expressed human liver cytochrome P450 3A4 catalytic activities by coexpressing NADPH-cytochrome P450 reductase and cytochrome b5, *Eur J Biochem*, **207**, 109–116.

Pompon, D., 1988, cDNA cloning and functional expression in yeast *Saccharomyces cerevisiae* of beta-naphthoflavone-induced rabbit liver P-450 LM4 and LM6, *Eur J Biochem*, **177**, 285–293.

Pompon, D., Louerat, B., Bronine, A. and Urban, P., 1996, Yeast expression of animal and plant P450s in optimized redox environments, *Methods Enzymol*, **272**, 51–64.

Pritchard, M.P., Ossetian, R., Li, D.N., Henderson, C.J., Burchell, B., Wolf, C.R. *et al.*, 1997, A general strategy for the expression of recombinant human cytochrome P450s in Escherichia coli using bacterial signal peptides: expression of CYP3A4, CYP2A6, and CYP2E1, *Arch Biochem Biophys*, **345**, 342–354.

Rendic, S. and Di Carlo, F.J., 1997, Human cytochrome P450 enzymes: a status report summarizing their reactions, substrates, inducers and inhibitors, *Drug Metab Rev*, **29**, 413–580.

Rettie, A.E., Wienkers, L.C., Gonzalez, F.J., Trager, W.F. and Korzekwa, K.R., 1994, Impaired (S)-warfarin metabolism catalysed by the R144C allelic variant of CYP2C9, *Pharmacogenetics*, **4**, 39–42.

Rochat, B., Amey, M., Gillet, M., Meyer, U.A. and Baumann, P., 1997, Identification of three cytochrome P450 isozymes involved in N-demethylation of citalopram enantiomers in human liver microsomes, *Pharmacogenetics*, **7**, 1–10.

Ronis, M.J.J. and Ingelman-Sundberg, M., 1999, Induction of human P450 enzymes: Mechanisms and implications, in Wolf, T. (ed.) *Handbook of Human Toxicology*, Marcel Decker, pp. 239–262.

Ronis, M.J.J., Lindros, K.O. and Ingelman-Sundberg, M., 1996, The CYP2E Subfamily, in Ioannides, C. (ed.) *Cytochromes P450: Metabolic and toxicological aspects*, pp. 211–239, New York: CRC Press.

Schneider, A., Schmalix, W.A., Siruguri, V., de Groene, E.M., Horbach, G.J., Kleingeist, B. *et al.*, 1996, Stable expression of human cytochrome P450 3A4 in conjunction with human NADPH-cytochrome P450 oxidoreductase in V79 Chinese hamster cells, *Arch Biochem Biophys*, **332**, 295–304.

Shimada, T., Yamazaki, H., Mimura, M., Inui, Y. and Guengerich, F.P., 1994, Interindividual variations in human liver cytochrome P-450 enzymes involved in the oxidation of drugs, carcinogens and toxic chemicals: studies with liver microsomes of 30 Japanese and 30 Caucasians, *J Pharmacol Exp Ther*, **270**, 414–423.

Shimozawa, O., Sakaguchi, M., Ogawa, H., Harada, N., Mihara, K. and Omura, T., 1993, Core glycosylation of cytochrome P-450(arom). Evidence for localization of N terminus of microsomal cytochrome P-450 in the lumen, *J Biol Chem*, **268**, 21399–21402.

Simula, T.P., Glancey, M.J. and Wolf, C.R., 1993, Human glutathione S-transferase-expressing *Salmonella typhimurium* tester strains to study the activation/detoxification of mutagenic compounds: studies with halogenated compounds, aromatic amines and aflatoxin B1, *Carcinogenesis*, **14**, 1371–1376.

Truan, G., Cullin, C., Reisdorf, P., Urban, P. and Pompon, D., 1993, Enhanced in vivo monooxygenase activities of mammalian P450s in engineered yeast cells producing high levels of NADPH-P450 reductase and human cytochrome b5, *Gene*, **125**, 49–55.

Urban, P., Cullin, C. and Pompon, D., 1990, Maximizing the expression of mammalian cytochrome P-450 monooxygenase activities in yeast cells, *Biochimie*, **72**, 463–472.

Urban, P., Truan, G., Bellamine, A., Laine, R., Gautier, J.-C. and Pompon, D., 1994, Engineered yeasts simulating P450-dependent metabolism: tricks, myths and reality, *Drug Metabol Drug Interact*, **11**, 169–200.

Wadelius, M., Darj, E., Frenne, G. and Rane, A., 1997, Induction of CYP2D6 in pregnancy, *Clin Pharmacol Ther*, **62**, 400–407.

Waterman, M.R., 1994, Heterologous expression of mammalian P450 enzymes, *Adv Enzymol Relat Areas Mol Biol*, **68**, 37–66.

Widersten, M., Huang, M. and Mannervik, B., 1996, Optimized heterologous expression of the polymorphic human glutathione transferase M1-1 based on silent mutations in the corresponding cDNA, *Protein Expr Purif*, **7**, 367–372.

Wild, D., Feser, W., Michel, S., Lord, H.L. and Josephy, P.D., 1995, Metabolic activation of heterocyclic aromatic amines catalyzed by human arylamine *N*-acetyltransferase isozymes (NAT1 and NAT2) expressed in *Salmonella typhimurium, Carcinogenesis*, **16**, 643–648.

Woosley, R.L., Chen, Y., Freiman, J.P. and Gillis, R.A., 1993, Mechanism of the cardiotoxic actions of terfenadine, *JAMA*, **269**, 1532–1536.

Wrighton, S.A., VandenBranden, M. and Ring, B.J., 1996, The human drug metabolizing cytochromes P450, *J Pharmacokinet Biopharm*, **24**, 461–473.

Villikka, K., Kivisto, K.T., Backman, J.T., Olkkola, K.T. and Neuvonen, P.J., 1997, Triazolam is ineffective in patients taking rifampin, *Clin Pharmacol Ther*, **61**, 8–14.

von Moltke, L.L., Greenblatt, D.J., Cotreau-Bibbo, M.M., Duan, S.X., Harmatz, J.S. and Shader, R.I., 1994a, Inhibition of desipramine hydroxylation in vitro by serotonin-reuptake-inhibitor antidepressants, and by quinidine and ketoconazole: a model system to predict drug interactions in vivo, *J Pharmacol Exp Ther*, **268**, 1278–1283.

von Moltke, L.L., Greenblatt, D.J., Duan, S.X., Harmatz, J.S. and Shader, R.I., 1994b, *In vitro* prediction of the terfenadine–ketoconazole pharmacokinetic interaction, *J Clin Pharmacol*, **34**, 1222–1227.

von Moltke, L.L., Greenblatt, D.J., Duan, S.X., Schmider, J., Wright, C.E., Harmatz, J.S. *et al.*, 1997, Human cytochromes mediating N-demethylation of fluoxetine in vitro, *Psychopharmacology (Berl)*, **132**, 402–407.

Yun, C.H., Song, M. and Kim, H., 1997, Conformational change of cytochrome P450 1A2 induced by phospholipids and detergents, *J Biol Chem*, **272**, 19725–19730.

Zuber, M.X., Simpson, E.R. and Waterman, M.R., 1986, Expression of bovine 17 alpha-hydroxylase cytochrome P-450 cDNA in nonsteroidogenic (COS 1) cells, *Science*, **234**, 1258–1261.

9 The Future of High Throughput Screening and Pharmacotoxicology

Michael Balls ECVAM, Italy

9.1 Introduction

I have had the privilege of reading most of the chapters in this book in advance of their publication. This has been an exciting experience at this relatively early stage of a new era in drug discovery, as impressive developments in instrumentation are being combined with new concepts in combinatorial chemistry and new levels of understanding of cells and the operations and interactions of their components at the molecular level.

Nevertheless, greatly impressed as I am, I also feel a certain unease, a degree of wariness, about the huge resources, and the huge expectations, being invested in the high throughput screening (HTS) approach. I cannot escape the thought that, breathtaking though progress in genomics and proteomics in recent years has undoubtedly been, the cells, organs and systems of the body will continue to hold mysteries for us for a very long while to come. They will remain our masters, and we must beware of the consequences of trying to apply too dramatically and drastically what we may mistakenly think is a sufficient understanding of them.

This chapter will therefore be in two parts – some reactions to what is presented in some of the other chapters, by authors whose knowledge, commitment and expertise in HTS is orders of magnitude above my own, followed by some cautionary thoughts based on my own experience and my conviction that we must also focus on improving the development and application of medium throughput screening (MTS) and low throughput screening (LTS) systems and strategies.

9.2 High throughput screening

The need for HTS to be extended from drug discovery to toxicology is emphasized by the editors of this book in their

> Breathtaking though progress in genomics and proteomics in recent years has undoubtedly been, the cells, organs and systems of the body will continue to hold mysteries for us for a very long while to come. They will remain our masters, and we must beware of the consequences of trying to apply too dramatically and drastically what we may mistakenly think is a sufficient understanding of them.

">

editorial (Atterwill *et al.*, 1999), and they see automation and efficiency as key elements in the development of the systems and strategies to be applied.

I hope that it will be possible to identify usable toxicity indicators for application in HTS, and I am glad that they also see the need for the extension of the emerging new technologies into the medium and low throughput modes. Nevertheless, and I say this as somebody heavily committed to *in vitro* toxicology and *in vitro* testing, we must not overlook the significance of complex interactions, not only at the cell and tissue levels, but also within and between organs and systems such as the endocrine, immune, and nervous systems. Also, many of the diseases which confront us are multifactorial in their origins and in their progression, and involve intricate interactions among genetic, individual lifestyle and environmental factors.

This theme is reflected to some extent in the chapter by Banks (1999), who focuses on the need for the identification of unique biological targets at the level of diseased cells. One of the keys to successful HTS, of course, will be demonstrating the selective interaction of candidate pharmaceuticals with these targets in ways which can be automated and reliably measured. This, in turn, leads to considerations of logistics and costs – and of savings. However, it is not possible to save until you know the costs, not only of the chemicals to be screened, the assay systems, the reagents, the microtitre plates, etc., but also of failing to detect what could have been detected. In other words, HTS in terms of compound throughput, degree of miniaturization, etc., will have its limits. It would be possible to have an HTS system which was the ultimate in speed, automation, efficiency and savings, but which never revealed anything worth following up. As one for whom the 96-well plate is almost a step too far, the very thought of the 9600-well plate appals me!

The chapter on cytotoxicity and mechanistic studies in HTS by Fry (1999) is much closer to my own experience, so, when I say that it is excellent and realistic, this opinion may have more value. I entirely agree with his first premise, that it will not be possible to identify all mechanisms of toxicity in any kind of HTS system. One of the problems with toxicology, as opposed to pharmacology, is that a particular screen can only tell us about a particular endpoint, whereas toxicology testing is ultimately about trying to detect the totally unexpected.

Nevertheless, I can also totally agree with Fry's second premise, that it will be possible to devise an integrated approach with a manageable battery of relatively HTS, or at

> One of the keys to
> successful HTS will
> be demonstrating the
> selective interaction
> of candidate
> pharmaceuticals
> with these targets in
> ways which can be
> automated and reliably
> measured. This leads
> to considerations of
> logistics and cost – and
> of savings.

least MTS, systems, so that valuable information on potential toxicity can be made available much earlier in the drug discovery/development process than at present.

This especially applies to *basal cytotoxicity* and *selective cytotoxicity*, although *cell-specific function toxicity* (Seibert *et al.*, 1996) will tend to represent the higher levels of organization and interaction I referred to earlier, which will need MTS and LTS approaches.

Fundamental to any HTS screening approach related to toxic potential will be exploitation of our increasing understanding of the stress response and of cell defence mechanisms (Kind, 1999), although care will have to be taken to ensure that the development and application of stress gene constructs and reporter systems will quantitatively and qualitatively reflect what could, and would be likely to, occur *in vivo*. This may be stating the obvious, and the thought applies no less to cells which have been genetically modified to contain certain metabolic pathways or to emphasize the role of apoptosis. However, it may also be that the obvious may sometimes not be stated sufficiently regularly.

I am glad that I did not have to think too deeply about pharmacogenomics when writing this chapter, but it was also something of a relief to see Farr and Burris' incisive analysis of the potential uses of molecular endpoints in safety evaluation, which is coupled with a number of warnings based on actual situations (Farr and Burris, 1999). It is indeed dangerous when assumptions are permitted to become dogma, and we must not underestimate the pleiotropic effects, not only of chemicals, but also of genes and patterns of gene activity.

It is against this background that the chapter by Todd *et al.* (1999) on branched DNA assays must be read, since the key to exploiting the undoubted possibilities afforded by toxicogenomics will necessarily be the scientific qualities of those who try to take these opportunities and how successful they are in doing so. It is in this context that I will first mention the word *validation*, which will appear frequently in the subsequent section of this chapter. Todd *et al.* have spelled out an elaborate and exciting strategy, and it will be interesting to see whether or not this approach (and a number of other approaches outlined in this book) will turn out to be relevant and reliable in practice.

As Fry (1999) has pointed out, detecting the potential for metabolism-mediated toxicity is a crucial aspect of toxicity testing in general. This applies when the test methods are based on *in vivo* or *in vitro* approaches, and whether they are based on MTS or LTS, as well as HTS, systems. Indeed,

It was also something of a relief to see Farr and Burris' incisive analysis of the potential uses of molecular endpoints in safety evaluation, which is coupled with a number of warnings based on actual situations.

success in the development of reliable and relevant genetically modified human and animal cells for predicting human drug metabolism will be essential, if the value of HTS is to be fully exploited.

Whether the use of non-mammalian cells to predict metabolism-mediated toxicity in HTS will be widely applicable remains to be seen, and Oscarson and Ingelman-Sundberg (1999) express some doubts about this in an excellent review of the current status of bacterial, yeast, insect and mammalian expression systems for drug metabolism enzymes.

The review by Kass and Jones (1999) on methods for assessing apoptosis is perhaps useful in its generality, but their link to HTS for investigating the potential toxicity of compounds need not be merely passive. For example, cells could be genetically modified so that a selective and readily demonstrable apoptotic outcome was linked to the tissue specific triggering of a particular gene or receptor. Conversely, of course, reporter genes could be used to provide readily detectable biomarkers for the triggering of apoptosis or other indicators of toxic effects.

9.3 The validation of HTS systems

Validation has been defined as the process whereby the reliability and relevance of a procedure are established for a particular purpose (Balls *et al.*, 1990). However, while there are various types of validation (Balls, 1992), and the independent management, selection of test materials and data analysis in a blind trial which characterize the formal validation of tests designed for regulatory testing would not be necessary in the evaluation of a procedure intended for in-house use within a pharmaceutical company, many useful lessons have been learned, which could usefully be applied in the development of tests for use in HTS systems (Balls and Fentem, 1999).

For example, the value of a test procedure depends on all of its component parts – on the relevance of the biological systems employed and of the endpoint measured, on the endpoint assay and its reproducibility, on the way in which a result is expressed, and on the quality of the prediction model used to convert the test result into an expression of the likely *in vivo* effect which is the focus of interest. All of these issues would have to be addressed, and must be kept under review, in the development and application of any HTS system.

Another important factor is the selection of the materials to be included in the training set to be used in the evaluation of the procedure, which is in turn dependent on the quality of the existing knowledge about those materials.

However, in the case of HTS, there is an additional factor. The ultimate commercial benefit will inevitably depend on the variety and quality of the chemicals which are screened. Some promising candidates will be found among the extensive stocks of chemicals already held by companies, but there will also be a need to create new chemical entities based on combinational chemistry and an adequate knowledge of the desired pharmacological activity.

For the prediction of toxic potential to be incorporated at an early stage in HTS, more will need to be known about fundamental mechanisms in toxicology and about common, pivotal events, which may lead to different kinds of toxic outcomes in different kinds of cells and tissues.

One encouraging development is emerging from the analysis of the Multi-Centre Evaluation of *In Vitro* Cytotoxicity (MEIC) scheme of the Scandinavian Society for Cell Toxicology. Fifty reference chemicals for which human lethal doses and lethal blood concentrations could be calculated were tested in one or more of 61 cytotoxicity tests in 29 laboratories (Ekwall *et al.*, 1998). It was found that rat and mouse LD50 values gave predictions of human lethal dosages which were only fairly good ($R^2 = 0.61$ and 0.65, respectively), whereas human cell lines gave R^2 values of 0.70 and more, which could be further improved if allowance was made for chemicals which would be likely to pass freely across the blood-brain barrier.

Thus, as Fry (1999) has pointed out, a strong case can be made for including a basal cytotoxicity test in HTS strategies for identifying chemicals likely to be toxic to humans.

Success is also being achieved in the integrated use of data from physicochemical tests, QSAR analysis and *in vitro* tests (Barratt, 1998), and 17 detailed recommendations aimed at increasing the value of non-animal methods for determining physicochemical properties, assessing toxicity, assessing metabolism and assessing permeability were recently made in the report of an ECVAM workshop on pharmacokinetics in early drug research (Leahy *et al.*, 1997). An ECVAM-sponsored study on *in vitro* models of the blood-brain barrier is about to begin, and a workshop is to be held on the use of Caco-2 cells as an *in vitro* model for Gl permeability studies.

Also impressive is the progress being made in developing a practical and integrated physicochemical/*in vitro*

One encouraging development is emerging from the analysis of the Multi-Centre Evaluation of *In Vitro* Cytotoxicity (MEIC) scheme of the Scandinavian Society for Cell Toxicology. A strong case can be made for including a basal cytotoxicity test in HTS strategies for identifying chemicals likely to be toxic to humans.

approach to biokinetics, as a means of predicting absorption, metabolism and distribution, and as a means of estimating the likely concentrations and half-lives of test chemicals and their metabolites in various target organ tissues, to make possible the more meaningful interpretation of *in vitro* test data (Blaauboer *et al.*, 1998).

Given that progress is also being made in the development of *in vitro* tests and testing strategies for immunotoxicity, neurotoxicity, embryotoxicity, haematotoxicity, hepatotoxicity, nephrotoxicity, etc., the day can be foreseen when it will be possible to select an appropriate and manageable battery of non-animal test methods for use in MTS and LTS strategies for candidate compound evaluation and selection. The creation of such strategies has been the aim of the ERGATT/CFN Integrated Testing Scheme (ECITTS) originated by Walum *et al.* (1992).

It can also be hoped that significant progress can be made in relation to the most expensive aspect of conventional animal-based toxicity testing, the two-species rodent bioassay for carcinogenicity. Some temporary reduction in costs might be achieved through the use of transgenic mice, although the need for the use of two species has itself been questioned, at least since the late 1970s. However, much more could be achieved through the validation and acceptance of cell transformation assays, such as the SHE cell assay (Aardema *et al.*, 1996), as was discussed at a recent ECVAM workshop. This could provide an MTS approach to replace the current LTS *in vivo* bioassay.

> Much more could be achieved through the validation and acceptance of cell transformation assays, such as the SHE cell assay, as was discussed at a recent ECVAM workshop. This could provide an MTS approach to replace the current LTS *in vivo* bioassay.

Two other points, one positive, one negative, are worth mentioning. Firstly, there is much current interest in biomarkers of exposure and effect (Bottrill, 1998), which could provide opportunities for linking activities in molecular toxicology, HTS and studies focused on target organ and target system toxicology. Secondly, I am concerned at talk of HTS approaches to the identification of chemicals with endocrine disruption potential. Whether such approaches would do other than cause immense problems for industries and regulatory authorities alike, would depend on a ruthless application of the principles of validation, and the objective and independent evaluation of their reliability and relevance in the real world.

This brings into sharp focus the need for establishing that testing is necessary, as a means of providing information which can be rationally applied and on the basis of which sound and sensible decisions can be taken. The test systems themselves must be demonstrably relevant and reliable for their stated purposes, no less in-house than in the regulatory arena, and they must be applied with great care and considerable skill. If the highest standards are set and can be met at all stages of the process, then HTS, intelligently used with subsequent MTS and LTS approaches, undoubtedly offers the prospect of the discovery, selection, development, manufacture and marketing of better, safer and more affordable pharmaceuticals.

References

Aardema, M.J., Isfort, R.J., Thompson, E.D. and LeBoeuf, R.A., 1996, The low pH Syrian hamster embryo (SHE) cell transformation assay: a revitalised role in carcinogen prediction, *Mutation Research*, **356**, 5–9.

Atterwill, C.K., Goldfarb, P. and Purcell, W., 1999, High throughput screening, new predictive technologies and genomics in toxicology – this volume, pp. 1–7.

Balls, M., 1992, *In vitro* test validation: high-hurdling, but *not* pole vaulting, *ATLA*, **20**, 355–357.

Balls, M. and Fentem, J.H., 1999, An update on the regulatory status of alternative methods, *Toxicology in vitro*, **13**, 837–846.

Balls, M. *et al.*, 1990, Report and recommendations of the CAART/ERGATT workshop on the validation of toxicity test procedures, *ATLA*, **18**, 339–344.

Banks, M., 1999, Automation and technology for HTS in drug development – this volume, pp. 9–29.

Barratt, M.D., 1998, Integration of QSAR and *in vitro* toxicology, *Environmental Health Perspectives*, **106**, supplement 2, 459–465.

Blaauboer, B.J. *et al.*, 1998, 13th meeting of the Scientific Group on Methodologies for the Safety Evaluation of Chemicals (SGOMSEC): alternative testing methodologies and conceptual issues, *Environmental Health Perspectives*, **106**, supplement 2, 413–418.

Bottrill, K., 1998, The use of biomarkers as alternatives to current animal tests on food chemicals, *ATLA*, **26**, 421–480.

Ekwall, B. *et al.*, 1998, MEIC evaluation of acute systemic toxicity. Part VI. The prediction of human toxicity by rodent LD50 values and results from 61 *in vitro* methods, *ATLA*, **26**, 617–658.

Farr, S., Dunn, R. and Burris, R., 1999, Toxicogenomics, this volume, pp. 43–65.

Fry, J.R., 1999, Cytotoxicity and mechanistic studies in high throughput toxicity screening – this volume, pp. 31–42.

Kass, G.E.N. and Jones, R.A., 1999, Methods for assessing apotosis – this volume, pp. 107–138.

Kind, C. and Hammond, T., 1999, Early toxic stressor genes – modulation and screening technologies – this volume, pp. 69–90.

Leahy, D.E. *et al.*, 1997, Pharmacokinetics in early drug research. The report and recommendations of ECVAM Workshop 22, *ATLA*, **25**, 17–31.

Oscarson, M. and Ingelman-Sundberg, M., 1999, Genetically modified cells to assess drug metabolism *in vitro* – this volume, pp. 139–170.

Seibert, H. *et al.*, 1996, Acute toxicity testing *in vitro* and the classification and labelling of chemicals. The report and recommendations of ECVAM Workshop 16, *ATLA*, **24**, 499–510.

Todd, M.D., Ludtke, D.N., Oshidari, F., Johnson, D. and Grushenka, H.I.W. 1999, The utility of branched DNA (bDNA) assays in high throughput screening – this volume, pp. 92–106.

Walum, E. *et seq.* 1992, ECITTS: an integrated approach to the application of *in vitro* test systems to the hazard assessment of chemicals, *ATLA*, **20**, 406–428.

Index

Numbers in *italic* indicate figures and tables.